WAKEFIELD PRESS

SOMEONE YOU KNOW

Born to Italian migrant parents and married with a young daughter, Maria Pallotta-Chiarolli teaches humanities in an Adelaide high school and works as a gender and equity project officer for Catholic Education. She is also a volunteer worker for the AIDS Council of South Australia. Maria is completing a master of arts degree in women's studies and has published several academic papers on issues of ethnicity, sexuality and gender. She has published poems and a short story in magazines and journals.

SOMEONE YOU KNOW

Maria Pallotta-Chiarolli

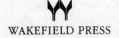

WAKEFIELD PRESS

Wakefield Press
PO Box 2266
Kent Town
South Australia 5071

First published October 1991
Reprinted November 1991

Edited by Jane Arms

Design by Ann Wojczuk
Cover illustration by Mitch Vane

Typeset and printed by Gillingham Printers Pty Ltd,
153 Holbrooks Road, Underdale, South Australia 5032

Cataloguing-in-publication data

Pallotta-Chiarolli, Maria, 1960-
Someone You Know
ISBN 1 86254 271 6
1. Pallotta-Chiarolli, Maria, 1960- 2. AIDS (Disease) –
Patients – Australia – Biography. I. Title

Creative writing program assisted by the Australia
Council, the Australian Government's arts funding and
advisory body.

*Part proceeds of the sale of this book
are being donated to the Bobby Goldsmith
Foundation of South Australia*

To Jon,
who said,

When it's all over,
tell them about me
so that they
may understand
someone they know

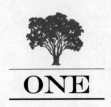

ONE

*You're neither unnatural, nor abominable,
nor mad; you're as much a part of what people
call nature as anyone else . . .*
Radclyffe Hall

1

I NEVER DID LIKE SYDNEY. As soon as I step off the bus I feel like climbing back on board. Passengers hurriedly collect their items without farewells. They disappear among the pedestrians jostling for room on the footpath. I feel as if there's a label on my back that says 'Frightened Foreigner'.

Only Sydney could do this to me. I like adventure. I do not mind being alone. Yet here, on this dirty footpath next to a congested road, I feel out of place and vulnerable. I sit on my suitcase, scanning the speeding traffic for the relieving sight of a red Mazda RX7 zooming by to scoop me up.

Half an hour later, there is still no red Mazda RX7. I'm beginning to feel irritable, aware how I must look to the grinning types who stare at me as they wander by. Wild black hair, black leather jacket, black leggings, black boots, and worried eyes in a solemn face.

Later, I lug my suitcase to the public telephones across the road. I lose my money in the first one, and the next two have been vandalised beyond use. I wait in a silent queue for the final booth. The man in front of me, large and grunting, shuffles up to the booth only to discover that his coins become stuck and refuse to dislodge even when his two heavy fists pound down on the contraption. He turns around and says, 'It's fucking full.'

My frustration kicks inside me. What a start to a holiday! From the moment I embarked on this journey, I knew something was out of place.

Perspiring in my leather jacket, I struggle back to the bus-stop. How unreliable of Jon. I had telephoned this morning and left a message about my time of arrival and where I could be picked up. What if something has happened?

I attempt to hail a passing taxi. One swerves dangerously to the kerb and the driver leans over the front seat, peering at me in silence. Through the open window, I hand him the scrap of paper on which the address is scribbled. Thank God it had buried itself deep in the pocket of my jacket. Without getting out of the car, he opens the back door and flicks a switch that opens the boot. I lift my suitcase in, close the boot, and sit down in the back seat.

'Just off the Cross,' he says abruptly, and not another word is exchanged as we speed away into the heart of Sydney. I wonder if this is the longest or shortest route, but I dare not ask. There's probably a switch that ejects nuisance passengers.

A few minutes and quite a few dollars later, he stops with a screech of brakes outside a multi-storey motel in a grimy street. He flicks the boot switch and sits silently, looking at the street, while I step out and retrieve my suitcase.

The motel looks dingy: the awning on the outside is dirty, the plastic plants in pots in the lobby are dusty and faded. There is no one at the front desk, no bell to ring. I walk to the lift and it rushes me noisily to the fourth floor. I rehearse my dramatic performance. The lift opens, and there is the wooden door. My fist rises and knocks sharply.

Jon smiles coolly at me. His neat moustache and combed, thinning hair annoy me. He's just finished breakfast, he tells me. Do I want some juice? Turning, he shuffles through the main room, which holds the dishevelled double bed, and steps into an adjoining alcove, the kitchenette. I follow, foolishly carrying my suitcase. I know that walk. I know those hunched shoulders.

I launch into an attack in which my words stumble over themselves, and my voice whines. Then I realise he isn't even facing me but squeezing oranges at the sink. The back of his neck, cleanly surrounded by a white shirt-collar, is the final display of insolence. 'Thanks very much!' I shout, and my eyes fill with tears.

Jon turns around, half oranges in his hands. His blue eyes shift from coolness to concern and back again but do not meet my own for long.

'You haven't even been listening to me.' I search his eyes.

He resumes his work while he talks. Yes, he'd got the message, but he'd been detained and by the time he was able to pick me up he assumed I'd be on my way to the motel. His shoulders look tense, his body is thin, elbows pointedly bony.

Something is very wrong. I feel he does not want me here.

Jon hands me my orange juice but doesn't look at me. He gulps his down and washes his glass, mutters something about tidying up, and goes to make the bed. I sit on a stool and peer out on the street below. It makes me feel dizzy. I look into the distance of rusty rooftops, dirty windows and faded advertisements that have long stopped fooling passers-by.

Silently, Jon returns to the kitchenette and begins to tidy the sink. He asks whether I've had a comfortable journey. The politeness cuts into me. I know that tone, but it has never been directed at me. Vaguely, I describe the bus trip, searching his face for signs.

I hand him my empty glass, which he leaves in the sink. 'Here I am in Sydney again. It hasn't changed,' I say, hoping to evoke a response I can understand.

'What did you expect?' he asks, looking at my suitcase.

What did I expect? Hugs and kisses, lots to say, laughter. But Sydney has caught us in its tentacles.

2

JON AND I entered the staff-room for recess, swapping stories about our assigned classes. I noticed the new teacher who had joined the school for the 1985 year sitting with colleagues. His name was Jim.

Tweaking his World War I Ace moustache, Jim thundered doom for the human race, lambasting us for our destruction of the environment, our overpopulation of the world. He took a passionate interest in philosophy, politics, events of the day. He knew so much that I wondered if his brain would burst. Raised by his mother, he didn't see what the fuss over gender roles was all about. Men and women were human beings, as good and as rotten as each other, he said. I warmed to Jim quickly.

I headed towards him, and Jon followed slowly. I made the usual introductions. 'We've met before,' Jim said.

'Oh yes, I know you, don't I?' Jon said politely, and then excused himself.

I missed the first signal. It was unlike Jon to be off-hand with new staff. Any new face was an instant target for twenty questions, some witticism, and a warm welcome. I was amazed how much people would tell him so soon. He would relate their life stories to me and any rumours worth remembering. 'I've got an honest face,' he'd tell me.

We'd been friends for two years. He was fun to work with, but I didn't always agree with what he said or how he said it, and I didn't think he always said what he really believed.

Uproarious laughter from a group of chairs around the low coffee-table: it was Jon's lunchtime revue, a welcome daily interlude in the classroom routine.

'A waste of protoplasm!' he said, and everyone laughed again. 'I stand at the front of that biology class and play spot the working brain cell. They play dumb so I don't expect them to lift their pens and scratch something intelligent on paper. So, what do I do? I launch into a provocative discussion of the reproductive cycle. Their eyes focus again; their hands, among other things, rise; and polysyllabic words spurt forth in an orgy of learning. Ten minutes later, I apologise to them for digressing and return to my original subject. But now they humour me with intelligent learning behaviour for the rest of the lesson.'

I sat down, crossing my feet on the coffee-table. Jon looked across. 'Most unladylike. No sense of decorum,' he said. Cheers from the stalls.

'But I'm not a lady, you see. And who set the rules for decorum?' Cheers.

'You're not a lady? I'd say you're quite a lady.' He pointed at my legs.

'I'm a lady because I've got legs?'

He swung his legs onto the coffee-table, his feet against mine, and rolled up his trousers to reveal his calves. 'Exhibit A. Exhibit B. Ladies and gentlemen of the jury, I rest my case. You may now decide who is the lady.'

'An excuse to show some skin, Jon?' I said it with a smile, but this side of Jon annoyed me.

'An excuse to get my bare legs next to yours,' and he winked mischievously. The crowd went wild.

Another lunchtime revue. I heard someone say, 'Here she comes. You're in for it now, mate.'

Jon bit into his sandwich and his eyes followed me.

I sat down. 'You carrying on again?'

'I just said feminism's the khaki crew-cut ideology.' The audience waited.

I sipped my coffee, refusing to be reeled in like limp bait. 'How many feminists do you know?'

'A few. More than enough.' Laughter.

'I'm a feminist.'

'You can't be a feminist. You're Italian.'

The audience gasped at his daring. I raised my eyebrows and laughed.

The bell rang. Colleagues began to leave. Jon remained seated. I stared at him. 'You weren't offended, were you?' he asked.

I shook my head slowly. 'But I wonder.'

'What do you mean?'

'You're too intelligent to believe all that bullshit.'

'It's fun, and you handle me well. I've never known an "ethnic minority person" quite like you.'

'And how many "ethnic minority persons" have you known?'

'Not many.' He grinned. 'Not closely anyway. I had a Seventh Day Adventist, Anglo-Saxon upbringing.'

'Well, I'm not unusual. I live in two cultures, drawing on, negotiating with each, and discarding what I don't like. I live in many worlds and I love it. You're an outsider. That's why you find me weird. You lump us all into one box. There's diversity in any subculture, Jon. The boxes we make for ourselves are very different.'

Jon smiled. 'So, blinded by stereotypes, I don't know you.'

I nodded.

'I should get to know you before I talk about you.'

I clapped my hands. 'You got it.'

He looked at me intently before brushing crumbs off his shirt. 'Back to the classroom.' He walked away, his head bowed, hands in pockets, shoulders hunched, feet shuffling.

It was the end of a busy day at work, and Jon was entertaining again in the staff room. 'You could tell he was – the way he minced his steps, the limp wrist.'

'Who are you raving on about now?'

'The guy, sorry gay, who was here to run that science conference.'

'How do you know he was gay?'

'You can pick a faggot.'

'And how many gay men do you know?'

'None that I know of.'

Jim came in and joined the sparring match. 'Do you know gay men, Maria?'

'Yeah, I have friends who happen to be gay.'

Jon sipped his coffee, watching us.

'What are they like?' Jim asked.

'Green, with three arms and one eye.'

'Seriously.'

'Diverse. One of my gay friends is Italian, so he'd be very much like me if you're into classifying.'

'Doesn't it worry you? Two men having sex?'

'What right have I got to tell anyone who to have sex with? Anyway, there's so much more to people that's important.'

'What about your religious beliefs?'

'My God says we should love one another, not judge, or condemn. Who am I to deny someone else's opportunity for love? I think we label gay men and lesbians through fear and ignorance.'

Jim cheered. 'We've all got the same red blood beneath our thin skins. Ain't that right, Jon?'

Jon gulped down the rest of his coffee. 'The issue doesn't interest me. I was just pointing out how effeminate some gay men are.'

'And so are some straight men,' I added. 'But what do you mean by effeminate? I'd say some gay men are more sensitive because of the shit they have to put up with. And some refuse to put on a big macho act like many straight men do. Poofter-bashers might be insecure about their own sexuality.'

I stared at Jon as I spoke. Everyone was waiting for Jon's reply. He glanced at me. 'Some would have to put up with an awful amount of shit, wouldn't they?' He left, head bowed, feet shuffling, shoulders hunched.

We all had slightly different versions of the life Jon led away from school before the time he came back for the 1984 school year sporting an engagement ring. She was from Adelaide but had lived in England for some years. Later, his engagement had been broken and she had gone to Sydney. Jon had spent weeks comparing marriage to mouse-traps.

Jim and I were sitting in the staff-room after school. It had been a difficult day for him; students were putting him through initiation rites. Jon offered his encouragement, relating some of his stressful experiences. 'So a student climbed through your classroom window! I had students hiding in closets!' Jon and Jim looked at each other and laughed. I didn't think it was so funny.

'Who would've thought such keen kids from Avondale'd be in the front lines?' Jim said, smiling warmly.

Jon rose. 'Got to go.'

'Going out, are you? Who is it tonight?'

'A buxom beauty.'

Jim snorted. 'You sex-starved bastard. Don't do yourself any harm!'

'A sexist bastard,' I said. 'A lady's man, eh?'

Jim roared, pulling at his moustache. 'He always thought he was a real man. Surfboard under his arm. Carefully oiled tan. Golden locks.'

'Well, let me go and perform my manly functions.' Jon grinned and raced out.

'What was he like at college?'

'When I arrived at Avondale, he was a second-year, one of the 'old hands'. Part of the group, very witty, but also very concerned with the spiritual in life.'

'Tell me more.'

'He was immaculate. Hair exact. He had a lot more of it then. Good clothes, neatly groomed moustache. Most of us were total scruffs.' Jim scratched his beard. 'Haven't changed, have I?' He leaned forward. 'He had a great reputation with a canoe, mainly in white water. Whenever he went down to the creek, off came his shirt and we reckoned he combed the hairs on his chest.'

I laughed.

Jim ran a finger along the arm of his chair. 'Who should

turn up as my biology prac supervisor? He was huge fun and taught us a lot. We became friends. In a smelly lab surrounded by dead cane toads.

'He asked me if I'd like to be in the support crew on a canoe trip to the Barrington River. Jon led the main assault group, going down the most inaccessible part of the river, almost a death trap. I bummed a ride on a canoe for a small section. I won't forget it. We were thrown out within minutes, then spurted down a mass of rocks and foam. I managed to crawl ashore some way downstream.

'No one was killed – just! One went under tree roots and barely escaped alive. Another was trapped against boulders with only his face above water and had to be rescued. Another two were flung over a waterfall after their canoe broke in half.

'We were all wrecked, tired, cold. All except you know who; he came sailing up, hair in place, with a big cheesie grin on his dial.' Jim sighed. 'I've missed the fun and unpredictability that made him one of me mates. He hasn't had it easy. His humour and his rebellion against the church got him into trouble, but he's come through.'

'Jim told me a lot about you,' I said to Jon the next day. 'You were quite a hero.'

Jon shrugged. 'It's a small world, isn't it?'

Jon invited me to his place. 'I've got myself a puppy that I'd love you to see. He's a gorgeous creature. A strange cross between German Shepherd and Husky needing all the love he can get.'

'I don't like dogs.'

'You've written him off already!'

He had built himself a replica of a Swiss chalet, incongruous between brick veneer houses. It was beautiful but painfully self-conscious. The garden was clipped and quaint, rows and rows of purple and white flowers, measured squares of lawn. The interior was inviting, with lace curtains and an open fireplace, an antique cuckoo clock, and an oak kitchen; upstairs, a balcony and two bedrooms. For over a year, he had talked about a friend who paid rent. I was never told his name. Now, I saw his motorbike in the driveway, his jeans and t-shirts strewn over the bed. Jon shrugged at the mess. 'One room I have no jurisdiction over.'

'You sound like a parent.'

I imagined a tall, hefty fellow clomping down the wooden stairs in thick black boots. Later that afternoon, I met Kevin. He was young, pale, delicate-looking, with spiky brown hair and attractive eyes. He didn't seem to want to say much. Jon told me that Kevin was a nurse and worked odd shifts, and then disappeared into the kitchen.

I tried to make conversation. Kevin remained kneeling on the carpet, avoiding my gaze, stroking the puppy he'd brought in from the laundry. 'This is Sven – Svengali. He'll bring some magic into my life,' Jon said. 'Conjure up witches, like you.'

'You spoil him,' Kevin said.

Jon looked at me, waiting for my assessment.

'He's cute, actually.'

Jon steered the conversation between the three of us expertly: Kevin hoped to live in Sydney, Jon liked Sydney but preferred to live in Adelaide. I told them Sydney frightened me.

'Jon's playing a synthesiser at this morning's assembly,' a workmate told me as we lined up our classes outside the hall. 'His own composition. Didn't know he could play.'

Alternately brooding and triumphant, melancholy and joyful, his music flirted and then hid behind chords. Jon never looked up, a faint blush on his cheeks and neck.

It ended quietly, like a sigh. There was a hush, then a crescendo of applause and cheers. Jon shuffled awkwardly to the back of the hall, head lowered, hands in pockets.

I sat on the teacher's desk, my throat dry from talking.

Students raced outside at recess. Why didn't any of them stop to ask me questions? I had just spent forty minutes reading and interpreting T. S. Eliot's 'The Love Song of J. Alfred Prufrock' and now they all rushed out eager to eat. Weren't they hungry for emotional or spiritual food? A few had said Eliot was depressing, weird.

I began to arrange my books. 'Great stuff, miss,' and there was Jon. 'I heard your voice through the wall.'

'I hope you found more meaning than some of these students.'

'They're too young. Eliot was brilliant, wasn't he?'

'Yeah, one of my favourites.'

'He's one of my mine too.' Jon sat on the desk, picking up my anthology of Eliot's poetry. 'I can identify with so much of what he wrote. Especially Prufrock.' He leafed through the book until he found the poem. 'I feel like Prufrock sometimes: restless, afraid, misunderstood.' Standing, he looked back at me. 'Sorry. Ridiculously morbid. Let's go to recess.'

I locked the classroom. 'You should've been an English teacher, Jon.'

'I like biology too much.'

The spell was broken. His audience was waiting. But as he turned the door-knob to enter the noisy staff-room, he turned to me. 'T. S. Eliot was my great uncle. Small world, isn't it?'

During the Easter school holidays, Matteo rang. He was in Adelaide, glad to be away from work in Mount Gambier where he was a local radio DJ. He was a good friend – we'd spent rollicking university days together – who meandered successfully between his Italian and gay identities. Sometimes, he'd reveal some traditional ideas about gender. Even after I married, he'd look at me with consternation if I was out with male friends. 'It's not really done,' he'd say.

'Look who's talking!'

He related the latest rounds of social gatherings and

gossip. 'I met a friend of yours at a party,' he said, his voice deeper. 'He works with you. Jon's his name.'

'Oh Jon. Yeah, we're quite good friends. He's really popular at work, keeps everyone laughing. What did you think of him?'

'He seems okay. Wish he had more hair on his head.'

'How did you get to be at the same party?'

'I tagged along with a straight friend.'

He didn't mention Jon again.

Back at work, behind Jon in the queue for coffee, I said, 'You know that friend I told you about? Matteo? He says he met you at a party.'

Jon turned around, smiling, searching my eyes. 'That's right. Small world.' He reached for a paper cup, steadily heaping spoonfuls of coffee and sugar. 'We exchanged some interesting tips on how to handle you.'

3

DINNER was a spicy Italian pasta dish. Jon glowed with warmth. Even when Rob and I queried the authenticity of his cooking – the tomato sauce from a glass jar – he didn't break out into racist jokes. He smiled and reflected on his love of Italian food, 'reminiscent of peasant camaraderie' he had found even in the 'teeming cities' of Italy.

Rob and Jon liked each other. They shared similar interests – photography and medical developments – and the same concern over thinning hair.

Rob said, 'Thinning hair is a sign of high testosterone levels, of virility. Isn't that right, Jon?'

'Then, Maria's in the sacred presence of two blonde Adonises.'

I sipped more wine. 'But one's too fat and one's too thin.'

They compared body weights. Jon wanted to put on muscle, Rob wanted to lose fat.

I listened as they talked about the houses they each wanted to build, compared ambitions. They rarely had an opportunity to get together. Two of my favourite men.

'You two have a very unusual relationship,' Jon said suddenly, drawing me back into the conversation.

'When you're married to Maria, nothing's routine,' Rob said.

Jon pushed his chair back, stood up and said, 'I'd like to show you my special photo album. We'll have some more wine.'

He appeared with champagne and we settled ourselves on the balcony around the wooden table, looking out at the lights of suburbia and the thoroughfares down the valley. The cool breeze touched our cheeks.

Jon opened the album. 'My parents.' He described them. They moved to Sydney to live in the Avondale Seventh Day Adventist community, strong believers. I noticed Jon resembled his father: small round head, wispy hair, small frame, gentle blue eyes. The mother: hair tied back neatly, small eyes, square shoulders, staring at the onlooker. 'They were good parents according to traditional rules. My father was a workaholic; my mother directed us with a firm hand. I have three sisters. One is doctoring the poor in Africa and has a couple of kids. She's kept her faith and made it work for her. My other sister is edging nervously towards the end of a dry marriage in Western Australia. I remember she was such a carefree girl. But children and monotony and a sense of inferiority have somehow stifled her. My third sister is somewhere in England.'

Jon sat back. 'I guess that's why I find your family set-ups so interesting. My parents meant well, but they drew this invisible barrier between themselves and their offspring: no earthy communication, cool and controlled, none of the passion of Mediterranean families.'

Pages turned. 'My college friends.' He described life at Avondale College, with its rock-climbing expeditions, athletic competitions, surfing and car rallies. 'Most of my friends are married now. Most have lost contact with their religion, not connecting to its self-denying nature. They want to dance, drink. The women want to wear the sorts of clothes you wear without being branded Jezebels. But most have kept the important values.' Jon paused. 'My girlfriend.' A soft-focus photograph of a girl smiling away from the camera. 'The girls liked me.' Jon smiled sheepishly. 'But this one was special. I think it's because I had sex with her. But she was interested in him.' On the opposite page, a tanned youth leaning against a surfboard, a smile creasing his face, blonde wisps of hair falling over his eyes. 'My best friend.'

Jon's hand hovered over the two images. 'We were a threesome.' He paused.

I waited for his next words. They arrived quietly. 'Do I dare disturb the universe?'

I smiled.

'You see, I loved her. But she loved him, and I loved him too.'

We were still looking at the tanned surfie and the blonde girl.

'By the time I was nineteen, I cared for him more, and that worried me. It was a mortal sin to lust after your own sex. But I loved him. So I had sex with her, to console myself with my functioning masculinity, and I became a Don Juan. We'd go swimming at Manly, muck about in the water. I ached for any excuse to touch him. I'd yearn to be alone with him, contrived situations so she wasn't with us, and I'd tell her I'd marry her someday if he didn't.

'She told me she was pregnant, that it was mine, and told my parents immediately. So much pressure. For the first time in my life, I decided to experiment with honesty and face the backlash. My experiment failed. I told her I'd be a good father to her child but that she deserved to know how I

16

felt. She raged in disgust and despair. How could she give her child a faggot for a father?

I rushed to him. I told him I loved him. He laughed, callously. 'I'm not queer,' he said, backing away. 'I've been fucking her too, mate.'

'I promised to take care of her and the child, but she had decided something else. 'It can't be yours! It won't be yours!' I remember her screaming.

'Soon after the child was born, she got engaged. I've only seen the little boy once – small, blonde, shy. He looked at me with my blue eyes.'

Jon paused. 'I tried to talk to my parents. Explain what I was, how I felt, and I guess, considering their beliefs and community structure, they did well. My father walked away from me, not wanting to know, reciting comforting religious verses under his breath. Later, he said he never wanted to hear me mention that word again in his house. I was his son and always would be, but the other thing was not to be given a voice. My mother held out her bible. She wanted me to read the preachings on homosexuality. I wanted to read her the words about love and acceptance. She said she'd pray for me. My sisters understood, and promised to love me.'

Jon gulped down some champagne. 'I realised from that time that this dilemma would evoke painful responses.' His eyes shone in the light. My hand closed over his. It was icy cold, the knuckles sharp. His fingers turned and folded around my hand. 'I've always thought I'd make the perfect gay Prufrock.' Jon looked into the night sky. 'There's more.'

'Let's have it then,' Rob said with mock grimness. 'We're ready.' He made to turn another page of the album.

Jon laughed as he brushed Rob's hand away. 'No, they're my deeds, my life. I'll turn the pages.'

He continued to piece his life together: leaving home, travelling overseas, relationships forming and falling apart. 'I often felt I was drowning in self-hatred, and then I'd struggle to swim, and I discovered self-dignity and self-acceptance. All the while, I was carving this puppet figure, you know what I mean, Maria, the cheeky but acceptable disguise.'

There was a photo of a class group on an excursion to the beach. Against the blue sky and blue sea, youths squinted in the sun. Jon pointed to one student on the edge of the group. He was plump, squeezed into a dirty-white t-shirt. 'This is Robbo. He hates this photo. He's quite stunning now, and thinking of getting married.'

Jon's story took another twist. 'I taught him here in Adelaide at the Adventist school. He always seemed lonely, needing to talk. So he'd hang around after class. We became friends – nothing sexual, nothing indecent. But rumours of sexual indecency began to grow, particularly after he came with me on a couple of photographic expeditions. I was called into the principal's office. What should I say? I was a respected member of staff, making professional contributions and toeing the religious line. My private life was clean.

'The principal had seemed reasonable, modern. Yes, he believed I was gay – he'd always thought so, he said. No, there must be more to this student-teacher relationship. He had no option but to request my resignation. Robbo was changing: he was more outspoken, rebellious, and I was a homosexual. A mortal sin. I remember he called it a "distasteful" issue.'

Jon shook his head. 'I soon found I had fewer friends than I thought. I went overseas where I did some crazy things. I turned my gayness into some sort of protest. I tried to enjoy the controversy, thrive on people's reactions to my exaggerated behaviour.' He ran a finger along his champagne glass.

'I came back to Adelaide and found myself owning a carpet-cleaning business. I was really cleaning out myself – and leaving a bit of a vacuum. I wasn't teaching, not giving anything of myself. I applied for a position at the Catholic school in this neighbourhood and got it. You met me there.

'I'd met a shy young man at a party who heard me talk

about my new job and told me he was an ex-student of the school. We fell in love.'

'Kevin,' I said.

'Yes. He was nineteen then. I was twenty-four.' Jon stretched out his right hand. 'We made our own vows three years ago. Since then, I've felt that things have fallen into place, but I worry. Do you understand me better now?'

'I can see why you lead a double life.'

Jon closed his photo album and traced patterns on the leather with his forefinger. 'At least you and your migrant families are considered socially useful. I'm a scourge. If I'm honest, I get crucified. The Italian philosopher Gramsci once said he functioned with "Pessimism of the mind, optimism of the will". That's how I live.'

Jon topped up our glasses. 'Jim knows it all. The first thing he said when we were alone was "G'day ugly", a standard Avondale greeting.

'Your friend Matteo's taken a fancy to me. I didn't know what he'd said to you. He kept urging me to tell you, but the last thing I wanted to do was to lose your friendship. So I've taken a risk, told myself that, if it failed, I'd move on from the school back to Sydney.'

'Jon, we'll stand by you.'

Jon nodded and smiled. 'You're full of life, you two. You see everything so simply, perhaps too simply sometimes. I don't want to become a burden.' Jon turned to me. 'I'm asking you to play along with my games, be the butt of some of my jokes when I need out.'

'So long as I can keep having you on about all that macho hype.'

Jon leaned over and kissed me.

4

JON SHOWED ME the newspaper article in the real-estate pages. He'd agreed to let a journalist write about his house. 'Read what it says about Kevin.'

I read the brief mention of a boarder who paid rent. 'He's furious,' Jon told me. 'After all, he had a hand in putting it together, and there's no acknowledgement of what he means to me. But what would they have done with the real story?' He made a fist with his right hand, screwing up the article as he did so.

As 1985 raced ahead, we were both building the houses of our dreams. Jon and Kevin flaunted the plans of their two double-storey townhouses next to their double-storey house, duplicating the European chalet style.

For two weeks at the end of the year they moved in with us. They would rent the house across the road from us when they returned from their holiday abroad.

Matteo arrived, dashed into the bathroom and called me on the pretence that he couldn't find a spare towel. A recent admirer, who was standing at the front door, had driven him all the way from Mount Gambier in the hope that Matteo would reciprocate his affection. Matteo grabbed me. 'Don't invite him in!'

When the fellow had gone, dejected, I blew up. 'You got this guy to drive you to Adelaide on false pretences. What if someone did that to you?'

Matteo laughed. 'They don't! I don't give them the chance. Maybe he'll learn not to be so gullible. Anyway, I made no promises.'

'You can be so callous!'

He apologised, encircling my waist. 'Don't be mad. I know I'm selfish, but I've only got a few days, and I don't want him round. I've come to see you guys, and catch up with your neighbour.'

I smiled and hit him lightly. 'That's it, isn't it?'

Matteo didn't stay long. Jon and Kevin had reconciled their latest differences over the building project and had resumed it with energy. Matteo managed to charm the same romantic into driving him back to Mount Gambier.

When Jon heard that, he chuckled and called Matteo a tart. 'I need a stable relationship.' He leaned against my verandah post. 'I'm worried that I'll lose Kevin. I was in my prime when I met him – mid-twenties, a skier's tan. Now I'm begining to lose my confidence: hair's thinning, bald spot enlarging, wrinkles scratching themselves into my skin, and he's beginning to talk about his dreams. I keep trying to entice him to share my life – the annual international trek, better houses. He's starting to resist my current, using the independence I encouraged in him against me.'

Jim called me over. 'Hey, some folks around here are beginning to wonder about you and Jon.'

'You're kidding.'

'He never stops talking about you.'

'What do you think, Jim?'

'I know you're just the best of friends. Others are wondering.'

'I never realised what diversity existed in an ethnic culture,' Jon said one evening after a party at my place. 'You for instance,' and he pointed his finger. 'You're so typically Italian, your talking hands, your flocks of family. But you're so different. You speak with an educated Aussie accent. You hang around with all sorts. You hate some Italian traditions, but you hate some Australian ways too. You refuse to be categorised. You're a feminist, and you won't be caught dead without make up. You're married and haven't a clue about so-called wifely duties and responsibilities. You're suburban, rustic and a fringe dweller all at once. We're a couple of chameleons, changing colours to survive.'

He'd walk in, sit down, and fold his hands. 'I'm here to

continue my anthropological study. Carry on. I need to observe you in your natural habitat.' Then he'd summarise his findings. 'Rellies and friends! There's always someone, whether you need a plumber to fix your toilet or a friend to sit and listen to you for hours. We Anglos with our turned-up noses need long, hooked noses that hook onto each other. You two live in a railway station with people coming and going.'

Jon would pretend to take notes. 'Now, let's see. The house belongs to your parents. You pay no rent. Half a dozen people have keys to your place and come and go as they please. You have chickens in the backyard, wholesome eggs and the ultimate in garbage disposal. You have your father's vineyards on the side of the house for grapes and natural red wine. What do we Anglos have? Sterile lawn and a couple of marijuana plants.'

'Hey! Some Italians have marijuana plants too!'

'Yeah, but on what a grand scale. They establish themselves like hard-working migrants do. And what about their backyard wineries and slaughter-houses?'

Music reverberated through the smoke-filled disco where Jon and I danced and laughed with friends. A male stripper took over the dance floor. At the end of his performance, we found a quiet place to drink and talk. 'You're not fussed by this scandalous environment,' Jon said.

'No different from any nightclub. Nice people, sleaze-balls.'

'That guy is staring at you.'

I followed Jon's gaze. A friend's brother was trying to hide behind his male partner. 'This is the only thing I hate. Coming here and making someone feel uncomfortable.'

'Go and talk to him.'

The hesitancy and fear in Rino's dark eyes begged me not to stay. He asked me when I'd be seeing his sister again. 'Tomorrow afternoon.' He bit his lower lip. He was only eighteen. 'It's all right, Rino. Don't worry.' I said goodbye and went back to Jon.

I told Matteo. He smiled. 'But you understand where we're coming from, don't you? It's harder for gay men and lesbians from Italian backgrounds to come out. I love my parents and don't want to hurt them. I say things like, "Of course I'll get married one day, I'm just waiting for the right girl." How can two old people who'd need to have the word "homosexual" explained to them ever come to terms with their gay child? They'd think it was something we'd picked up from Australian friends. They've lived through poverty, war, hunger. They come to a country where they have to start again in everything. They make a thousand sacrifices for the kids they cherish. After all that, I haven't got it in me to break their hearts. Some might handle it. Your parents don't seem to be fussed with me at all. But what if I was their son?'

'What if Tony or I was gay?' I asked my parents.

We were seated around their dinner table on a Sunday evening, my brother and his girlfriend Eva, on one side, Rob and me on the other, sharing my mother's Sunday banquet, and the usual animated conversation.

We'd been talking about Jon and Kevin renting the place across the road. My parents thought they were *bravi*. After all, they were our friends, and judging by the way they kept an eye out for me when Rob was away they must be decent. 'But they're too skinny,' my mother had said, heaping more pasta on Rob's plate. 'They'll get sick. Why don't you cook them some nice Italian meals?'

'She hardly cooks for me, Mum,' Rob said. 'I don't think any of Maria's friendships extend that far.'

Mum lowered her cushiony frame into a chair and shook her head. 'I see Kevin at the hospital when he comes into the cafeteria for lunch. I fill his plate when the supervisor isn't watching. I do that with a lot of those young nurses. They're all so pale and sickly.'

I would often stand back and watch my parents talking to Jon and Kevin over the front fence, their cheerful voices carrying across the road. I was so proud of them. My father discussed his vineyard and winemaking with Jon, an interested listener, unlike his own children, who wouldn't drink his wine but bought sweet wines full of chemicals. My father's tall dark frame shadowed Jon's and his hands cupped a bunch of grapes. Jon selected one. My mother would invite them to come over any time and take eggs from the chickens because her daughter rarely cooked decent meals and they'd rot.

'Yeah,' Tony said, his deep voice blaring out defiantly. My brother enjoyed a good family debate. 'What if I was gay?'

Eva laughed her loud, infectious laugh and hit him. 'Oh my God, I can just imagine it. I reckon you'd be really butch!'

'Well, if that's the way God made you, what could we do?' Dad said. 'I'd feel sorry for you. It would hurt me to think you'd have to face so much trouble but – ' He shrugged, holding the palms of his hands to the sky. 'There's an old saying, "*Il mondo è bello perché è vario:* The world is beautiful because it is varied".'

'Has Matteo told his parents?' my mother asked.

I shook my head.

My mother sighed. 'I wish he could. They'd have to understand. But as a mother I can see how hard it would be. He's such a good-looking piece of manhood.'

We laughed at her description. 'You've always had a thing about good-looking men,' my father said. 'The first time you met Robert here, you embarrassed him by telling him he had nice legs. What about me?'

My mother grinned and raised her eyebrows at him. 'Eh, you're getting old now.' She poured him a glass of red wine.

'I still think you're a beautiful woman. Not like your daughter here.' Dad turned to Rob with a look of scorn. 'Tell me, what do you grab onto at night? She's all bones!'

'What an Academy Award performance,' I said at the end of lunch. Teachers were moving off to classes. 'You make me laugh so much. It's worse now because I know what's really going on. Although sometimes it makes me burn. Why is it all so necessary?'

'Maybe it isn't. I'm sure a lot of my friends would have no problem with what I am. But some would. Anyway, I really enjoy being the court jester. You get to tell some truths.'

Jon took my arm and steered me towards the noticeboard. He glanced around quickly before he spoke. 'I'm in high spirits today. Look!' I read an official statement from the Education Department that said people could not be fired because of homosexuality. 'Isn't that great? They'll never be able to fire me again as long as I behave myself on the job.'

Now and again, Jon took risks, sent out clues, and sat back almost wanting someone to piece them together. He began to invite more work colleagues over for 'gatherings'. Kevin would sometimes be present, behaving like the friend who shared the house. A new teacher called Michael who joined the staff made it easier. He had been an ex-student at the school and a friend of Kevin's. There was no need to pretend. He and his girlfriend Simone began to see a great deal of us outside school.

One evening, Jon suggested a group of us go dancing. He took us to a gay disco. Alarmed, I whispered, 'What are you up to? Do you know what you're doing?'

He smiled. 'I'm curious.'

Over a cup of hot chocolate in Jon's kitchen, after the others had left, I asked him why he did it. 'Playing silly games, I guess. Perhaps they'll put it all together. It was like a trial so I could listen to their verdicts. It was careless, but it was based on a lapsed moment of wishful thinking.' He looked into his empty cup.

'If they had said anything, I would've told them a few things about friendship and hypocrisy.'

Jon looked up and smiled. 'I'm sure you would. Hair flying, hands flying.' He leaned forward. 'Do you think they guessed?'

'No one said anything. They figure you're a man of the world who frequents trendy places where straights and gays mix. Some hadn't been to a disco for so long, they assumed they're all like that now.'

We laughed.

Wandering about the yard doing my early morning duty, I noticed a group of senior students huddled together near the fence. Smoko, I decided. I made my way over slowly, giving them time to disperse before being caught red-handed. But they stayed as they were. 'What's going on?' They were looking out onto the road, some distance to the left. They sniggered.

'Please move away from the fence,' I said.

They began to walk off. 'We're not doing anything, and it's not girls,' one of the leaders told me. He looked sideways at his mates.

'Go on! Tell Mrs Chiarolli!' his friends urged.

Just then, Jon walked by, bag in hand, nodded at me, greeted the boys, and made his way towards the staff-room.

'Tell me.'

More giggles. 'We were just watching him being dropped off by his boyfriend.' Loud guffaws. 'We were just wondering how he managed to score a good-looking guy like that.'

'What have we talked about in class? About labelling and gossiping?' I spoke steadily.

'We know,' the leader nodded. 'We're just mucking around. We stir him up about it to his face sometimes. He doesn't say he isn't gay, but he doesn't say he is.'

I wanted to say more. They wandered away, still chuckling. Sellicks Beach at night was peaceful. Jon had planned to take some year eleven students to spend two days and a night in a cave at the beach conducting some fieldwork. 'Come along,' he urged. 'I want these kids to experience the natural coastal beauty, the sounds of the ocean at night, the peace of starlight and an open fire, the warmth of human beings huddled together in a cave.' He lowered his eyes. 'Sloppy, aren't I?'

'Sounds blissful.'

'It'll be a good break for me. So many arguments lately over that bloody building; he's threatening to leave me to finish it all off on my own if I don't stop bullying. Yes, it really is my dream, this bourgeois obsession with a posh home in a posh suburb, warming arthritic knees in front of a fire and a shawl around my shoulders.' Jon laughed dryly. 'I'm not even thirty.'

So we went to the beach.

Some of our students dropped live crabs into boiling water over the campfire, their faces devilish in the light of the flames. Jon and I were horrified when we came back from the water's edge. Jon couldn't understand such cruelty. 'We need to respect life, even the lives of crabs. Their hard shells won't protect them from pain. Death comes to all of us. So does pain. Why force it on anything? We should all have a chance to die at peace with ourselves.'

His words seemed to echo in the still blackness outside the circle of our campfire.

Most of the students were ashamed and apologetic. They sat in groups talking in reverent whispers. One or two sniggered uncomfortably or cast scornful glances at Jon. By two in the morning, they were silent lumps in sleeping bags.

Jon tended the fire. 'What they did to those crabs. What they call each other if they dare to get too close. What would they do to me?'

I put an arm around his waist, and rested my head on his shoulder. The flames blurred in front of my eyes.

5

IN JUNE, 1986, Jon and Kevin moved into their house, the framed photos of overseas trips and the cuckoo clock given pride of place. They had spent weeks painting, paving, tiling, cleaning. The townhouses were up for sale.

One afternoon, we heard a sports car roar and honk outside. A rich red Mazda RX7 was throbbing in our driveway, sparkling in the sun, Jon at the wheel. Broad grins and bright eyes greeted us. Rob and I took a closer look. Although second-hand, the car, an impulsive buy, was in luxurious condition. Jon told me the car was a sign for Kevin that they'd be enjoying life like they used to.

By November, the optimism had gone. The Australian economy had gone bad. Real-estate sales had collapsed and no one seemed prepared to pay the prices for the townhouses. A new edginess crept into Jon and Kevin's exchanges.

One day, Jon left work at lunch-time. That evening, he rang wanting to see me. I found Kevin restless, Jon listless. 'The bank underestimated the economic situation when they allowed us to take such a risky step. The house goes up for sale in a fortnight. We move out this weekend.' Jon leaned against the stairs, fists deep in pockets. 'I really felt settled here.'

Kevin sat on the lounge. 'Look, it's too big anyway. And the whole scheme was a risk.'

'The bank backed us, Kevin. They told us to go ahead.' Jon's face tightened.

'We got sucked in. We should sell the whole bloody lot.' Kevin walked past us to the front door, tears in his eyes.

I wanted to call him in, but Jon had gone into the kitchen and poured tall glasses of wine for the two of us.

The furniture and sentimental pieces were re-arranged in a townhouse. Jon and Kevin watched strangers pacing about in their house. One auction failed and another was scheduled. 'All that bloody hard work,' Jon muttered.

'I told you it would be a gamble,' Kevin said. 'Why don't we move to Sydney?'

'Paul and his partner have just broken up,' Jon told me one Saturday morning as we watched potential buyers roaming about his house. His hands were deep in his pockets, his eyes anxious and sad. 'After so many years together and a successful business, that's it. A new lover.'

It cast a shadow over Jon and Kevin. They united in helping their friend, but they were barely surfacing. Jon was plagued by feelings of sexual inadequacy and ageing although he was only just turning twenty-nine, and the constant arguments were wearing him out. But he and Kevin would come together, vowing not to let it fall apart.

In December, they threw a housewarming 'to spite the evil Gods'. The house had finally been sold.

School ended for another year. Summer holidays stretched before us. Jon and Kevin were not travelling this year. No money. No enthusiasm. Jon and I sat on my balcony and watched Adelaide trees and roofs shimmer in the sun. The city centre looked like a ring of grey Lego blocks planted neatly by a child. 'Kevin uses going to Sydney as a threat, dangling it over my head. And he's going out with other friends.'

'Once he felt awkward with your teaching friends.'

'It's a bit of a cycle, isn't it? We all get our moment.'

We talked about relationships: how people outgrew each other, needs and directions changed. Love became a mill-stone, keeping two people breaking and repairing, travelling nowhere. 'I'm proud I helped create such a strong adult,' Jon said scanning the horizon. 'But the creation's revolting against his maker.'

In February 1987, Jon and Kevin decided to sell the second townhouse. 'It's time to rent,' Jon said bitterly, 'get back to a transient way of living. Kevin wants to move closer to the city.' He gazed at the walls he had painted, cleared his throat and opened the front door for the Saturday inspection.

It was Kevin's twenty-fifth birthday in April. Jon and Kevin had not yet moved out but, even as Kevin's plans and needs became more definite, Jon began to bargain. 'Maybe renting a nice place without any of the financial problems of ownership will revive us,' he said. 'Maybe it's all a passing phase. He needs time for himself, but he still needs me.' He organised a surprise birthday party.

Kevin rang a week later, asking to see me. When I arrived, Jon wasn't there. 'I want you to know the way things are.' He was anxious, finding it difficult to explain. 'I would do anything for Jon, always will, but I no longer want him as a lover. I'm grateful for all he's done, but I have to go it alone. Sometimes, I feel so claustrophobic, Maria. His expectations suffocate me. The more I step back, the more he imposes.'

His eyes filled with tears. 'I want to explore, take risks. But Jon is ready to settle down. He seems to be retreating into premature old age – two faggots sharing a house and a dog. When I met him, he was lively. I admire him for all he's done, but I resent him. I've been following him like a puppy, never really growing up.' Kevin winced. 'I know it's my fault too. I accepted it like this, you know, the teacher and the student. I'm so angry with myself that I can turn around now and hurt him. What am I to do? I want to be free.' He wiped tears of frustration from his cheeks. 'I wanted you to understand and help him through. I don't want us to lose our friendship.'

By June, Jon and Kevin were living in Unley in a lacework villa. Jon displayed the leadlighting and ornate ceilings.

'The landlord is Italian. He'd have to be one of your mob, wouldn't he?'

'Here comes another stereotype,' I said.

Sparring was refreshing. The lightheartedness showed Jon's renewed optimism. Kevin had decided to move in with him, and they had been united again in helping Robbo, who arrived one night shaking and crying. His wife had left him, Jon told me. She had a new lover, a worldly man. They'd gone to Sydney. The wildly beautiful woman who was going to give him confidence had gone.

Jon and Robbo drew together, two wounded soldiers.

Jon appeared in my empty classroom before school began for the day. 'You'll like this,' he said, his mouth curling bitterly. 'Kevin has an Italian lover who comes over and simpers after him. He's tall, with a shiny black mane and bulging muscles, and he laps up every syllable Kevin utters. He's everything I'm not. He puts Kevin on a pedestal like he used to do to me. But he'll soon tire of this brainless hulk.'

By the end of June, Jon and Kevin had moved twice. Kevin wanted to live in the city. He wanted Robbo to move in with him on the understanding that Jon would come too. They found a townhouse in Sturt Street that was spacious and classy. All three agreed it was an excellent place.

Only Jon intended to stay. Robbo was talking of Sydney. He was thinking of resuming his studies at the Adventist College. Jon encouraged him, but he was also sad. 'The two young pigeons want to fly the coop.'

'You've got to let go, Jon,' I said. 'You've had your opportunities to do things your way. You know they'll always be there for you.'

Jon smiled and hugged me. 'Thank goodness for one stable person.'

'Oh, so you don't really think I'm a crazy Italian woman?'

One cold day in late June, Jon came to work, his face drawn, his damp hair wispy, fists buried deep in pockets. We stood near a classroom doorway, away from other ears. The wind made our clothes flap. 'Kevin's leaving. He's got a position at St Vincent's in Sydney. He's told his Italian stallion it's all over. Hasn't said that to me.' His lips curled. 'He wants to go on with nursing and from there go to India. Wonderfully good soul, isn't he?'

I didn't know what to say. I understood his ambitions. A few months before I'd gone to the Royal Adelaide Hospital to have lunch with a girlfriend. She happened to work where Kevin was stationed. With pride and enthusiasm, he had shown me around. He spoke to patients with sensitivity. Their faces lit up as he approached, and they tried to keep him talking for as long as possible.

Jon's cynical laughter ended my reminiscence. 'Now that he's actually going, he's making all sorts of promises. He's like a guilty boy.'

'Kevin'll be leaving on July the sixth,' Jon sneered, 'after Independence Day. Are you going to fire cannons as you march out of Adelaide?' Kevin was packing books into boxes.

'I'll need a fanfare if I survive your whingeing!' They smiled at each other, intimate friends who'd shared more than could be shelved in some archive.

On the night before Kevin left, at the farewell party, Jon was the gregarious host, wandering from group to group, tossing out witty remarks and eliciting riotous responses. Jon and I managed some time alone in the kitchen before I left. He scraped left-overs from plates into a plastic bag with sharp strokes of a knife. 'I can't bear it,' he whispered. 'What will I do after he shuts the door? What will he leave me with?'

'You'll be okay. You're a survivor. It's not the end.'

'No.' He filled a glass with tap water and gulped it down. 'There'll be more to it.'

'I'll come over tomorrow afternoon.' I put an arm around his shoulder. 'We'll go for a walk or something. I have to help Maria prepare for her housewarming in the morning.

See? Things are working out well for her now. A new man. A new house. She'd never have seen herself this happy a couple of years ago. She was on the verge of suicide, remember?'

Rob and I drove home. I found myself crying.

The sun shone half-heartedly on a Saturday afternoon. I'd spent the morning in Maria's warm cottage kitchen doing more talking than preparing food for the evening's party. Her life had been a chaotic roller-coaster, but the track ahead was becoming smoother; she had worked at it.

I admired her strength, the resilience of her humour. 'So I told my father that I don't give a shit whether he thinks it's ridiculous to have a housewarming and not even be married. This is my bloody house. I want to warm it up and I don't give a fuck how many rellies are going to have heart attacks. They're the same ones who had the heart attacks when I went to uni, when I married a Pom, when I divorced him and decided to live alone. If they haven't died by now, they never will.' She talked rapidly and loudly. For quite a while now, she'd decided she'd be heard.

'How come your parents don't dish out all this bullshit? How come your Dad thinks I'm really great and my Dad's always threatening to kill me before I kill him? The old heart again, you know. My scandals are going to be the end of him.' She crunched into a carrot. 'But who do you blame? I can just imagine the hell he went through living with my grandmother. That woman has balls down there somewhere, I'm telling you.'

We burst out laughing.

'Anyway, enough. You say hello to Jon for me. Tell him I know what it's like. Being left alone after a relationship is shit. Tell him I almost did myself in after a bottle of strega and a crazy joyride in a car. Tell him it ain't worth it. He'll get through. I know that now for sure, and no matter how supportive you are, Maria, he's going to have to get through it himself. It's a real dark road.'

33

I knocked at his door in the quiet street. He opened it with a weak smile. The house was dim and the stale smell of cigarettes hung in the air. We sat and listened to music.

Jon leaned back in his old armchair, staring at the red and green lights dancing on the stereo, as Foreigner performed 'I Want To Know What Love Is'. His hands were folded together white-knuckled. I sat on the carpet leaning against his chair.

He sat forward, eyes bright in his pale face. 'I'm going to Sydney in a couple of weeks, in the next term holidays. I'll catch up with old friends. Why don't you come?'

Before I could reply, he grabbed my shoulder. 'We'll have a rage. I'll show you Sydney. Enjoy ourselves before it's too late.'

'Yes, I'll go with you. I'd love to.' Jon took my hand in both of his. 'Fantastic! I'll go over in the first week of school holidays and you come over in the second. I'll have a week to see what has happened – whether my love-life has really drowned – and then you come over and resuscitate me. We'll drive home together. Just think!'

'I don't want to get in the way. You might need that time to work a few things out.'

Jon's smile faded. 'I'd like you to be there, Maria. The break's been made, but I need to go and see it to believe it. I'll need you there. There are so many changes ahead and I'm scared.' He looked back to the red and green lights.

'Yeah, we'll rage, Jon,' I said quietly. I moved so that I could lean against his legs. He massaged my shoulder.

6

'SO WHAT WOULD YOU like to do?' Jon asks without enthusiasm, resigned to playing host to an unwelcome guest. I assure him I don't care; whatever he wants to do. He thinks for a moment, and then suggests a long walk: Hyde Park, the Harbour, the Opera House, the Rocks. 'Perhaps you don't feel up to it?'

'I'm fine.' I feel giddy: lightheaded from the bus, lack of restful sleep and tension, or all of the above. But I'll be the compliant guest until it's right to ask him what has happened.

We set off. The pavement occasionally liquifies beneath my feet; people seem to be running into me. Everything is bathed in a half light.

'I've booked another room for you. I realise I said we'd share, but I would really prefer my own room. I'll pay for yours.'

In Hyde Park, Jon suggests that he take a photo of me sitting on the edge of the fountain. 'So you can remember your holiday here.'

I set a smile on my face, but I keep my sunglasses on. I ask him to pose for me so I can photograph him, but he shakes his head and is about to move on. 'Why not?' I ask sharply. 'I want to remember my holiday.' My voice has a brittle edge. I hide behind the camera, pretending to focus, trying to see what he's really feeling. As he looks intently into the camera, I study his face. I zoom in on the set mouth and gaunt cheeks. He stares back.

We stop for lunch in a plaza and watch office men and women scoffing sandwiches. I'm not very hungry. I feed bits of bread to the seagulls. Jon takes a few bites of his sandwich and wraps it again. He looks around him, stands, and mutters that he needs to find a toilet. He walks away quickly, shoulders hunched, hands in pockets. I'm left alone feeding seagulls, trying to ignore the dizziness inside me.

Jon takes some time before walking back, wiping his mouth with the back of his hand.

We walk to the Harbour, gazing up at the frame of the bridge and its partner, the dirty-white Opera House. They're still and sombre.

Jon gazes out over the water lapping against the concrete embankment. Something has died in him.

'What's wrong?'

'What do you mean?' He glances at me before turning back to the water. He grips the rail.

'Why aren't you talking?'

'I'm giving you a rest.'

'You're not being honest.'

'I'm deceptive?'

'You're shutting me out, and you're not telling me why.'

Jon takes a few steps away from me, leans on the rail again. I move up alongside him. He points at the houses. 'You'd think that those clean walls and manicured gardens meant everything was under control.'

'What's happening? What can I do?'

He straightens up and gently pulls his arm away. 'You're asking too many questions.' He shuffles away.

I don't follow.

He turns around and shouts,' Let's go to Manly by ferry! A trip to Manly! My surfie adolescence!'

'Don't change the subject!'

Jon looks at the ground and slowly walks back.

'I think I know.'

'I don't think so.' He smiles wryly.

I grab his arm. 'Jon, I can't stand seeing you like this and not knowing what to do.'

His voice is weary. 'I can't help the way I look.' He blows out a nervous sigh. 'Let's go to Manly.'

Jon leans over the rail of the ferry. I lean against the edge of it too, but I'm looking at him. The gulls shriek and swoop.

'So what's wrong with me, Maria?' We've been walking along in silence, watching our shoes become swallowed in the coarse sand. We both have our hands in the pockets of our leather jackets; we look to our shadows as if those dark anonymous figures, one thin and bowed, the other surrounded by flying curly hair, hold the key to the cage around us.

'I feel you don't want me here – '

'True.'

'I'll go home.' Childish tears well in my eyes.

Jon kicks at a stone.

'I don't understand. You're frightening me.'

'Maybe you don't. You're very perceptive, but you've put two and two together and come up with three. I don't want to frighten you.'

'Whatever's going on, let me know if there's something I can do.'

Jon puts his arm through mine. We're nearing the promontory. 'Let's just walk a little longer.' I stoop to pick up a shell. I feel its grooves and the smoothness inside.

'I don't want you to know, but I need you to know. I don't want to burden you. Is it fair to hurl a grenade at you and expect you to hold it?'

We walk on. 'I've been feeling sick for a long time. Nausea, diarrhoea, but I didn't want to know.'

7

IN JANUARY 1986, Jon and Kevin returned to Adelaide from their European and American 'jaunt', rested and contented, to find me looking ill. I had a severe bout of stomach virus for three weeks.

Jon stroked my cheek. 'You look so pale and tired. You're not used to being sick, are you? You know, some people face those symptoms daily due to one thing and another.' He laughed. 'I bet you thought you were dying.'

I grinned sheepishly. 'It had crossed my mind once or twice. I told you I'm a wimp.'

'I've had a pretty good run in my life. I was born with a strong constitution.'

'You must've given me your wog,' he said a few weeks later. 'I feel awful.'

'I feel great now. Serves you right for always calling me a wog. You can have it now all to yourself.'

Throughout the year, as Jon and Kevin's relationship faltered and the building project crumbled, Jon became frequently ill. 'All this stress is making me very susceptible to gastro,' he said as he downed medications or held onto me as a wave of dizziness washed over him. 'I've got to get my love-life in order.'

Early in 1987, we went to a gay club where we found the music and atmosphere exhilarating. Jon and I danced, but his movements seemed mechanical, unlike his usual rhythmic style. He was breathing heavily and, after one song, he needed to sit down. The music pounded away while he wiped his forehead. We sat and watched Kevin laughing, talking and dancing. Every now and again, he'd glance across at Jon. At one point, he came over and berated him. 'Stop acting like an octogenarian and have some fun.'

'I feel very ill this evening.'

Kevin stared at him, touched his shoulder for a moment, and returned to his group. Jon looked at me. ' "I grow old –".'

'You're lucky I'm a nurse,' Kevin said. We were worrying about Jon's fainting spells. He'd missed work again, and I'd gone over to see him. 'What's your boss going to say if you keep taking days off?'

'I've got plenty of sick days left. I've never been so sick.'

'You're getting yourself all worked up about things. The past is the past. I'm still here. Lucky for you. You know, if I hadn't caught him as he fell in the shower, I'm sure he would've cracked his skull.'

When Kevin had left for night duty, I asked Jon to try to relax. 'This stress could kill you. You've got a lot of living to do, and you're letting it drag you down.'

Jon lashed out. 'Why was I dealt this hand of cards? I didn't fucking beg for them.'

His anger concerned me. There was a renewed venom and panic every time he got ill.

'What does the doctor say?'

'I'll end up with an ulcer, a stroke, a nervous breakdown. More pills, more liquid.'

'I'm so glad you're still around, Kevin. He really needs you.'

'But he's starting to manipulate me, trying to make me feel responsible. He says some weird things about being sick, like how he'll probably die before we know it.'

Jon emerged from the toilet. I hugged him. He felt limp and frail. He hadn't been at work for three days and hadn't eaten much.

'What's the use? I vomit it all out, and all I get is pills, the panacea against what's really hurting me.' He eyed Kevin.

'Oh, stop feeling sorry for yourself! I'm doing what I can to help you, but you have to snap out of this.'

Jon clicked his fingers. 'Like this, my darling?'

Kevin looked at me. 'See what I mean?' He glared at Jon. 'You're enjoying this. You're doing this to keep me here. Well, you're old enough to stand on your own two feet.'

Kevin went out soon after. I made Jon some weak camomile tea. 'It's a good old-fashioned remedy for everything from baby teething to kidney trouble in the aged. We Italians swear by it. I was raised on this stuff.'

'Does it cure everything?' Jon asked cynically.

'Well, you've joined the land of the mortals,' Jim mocked as Jon sat quietly at lunch. 'You're really sick, aren't you? God, we used to think you were beyond that. You're flesh and blood, after all.'

Jon put his untouched sandwich on the table and tried to smile. 'At least it's keeping me quiet. Now you can all get stuck into me.'

'But you're still going to Sydney for a holiday. You never

stop. You should spend those two weeks sleeping.'

'Being asleep is like being dead. No thank you.'

'I began looking for signs,' Jon tells me, the sound of the surf in the background. 'Night sweats, dizzy spells, mouth sores, loss of weight. I began to realise something was terribly wrong. Since the end of last year, a certain thought has been haunting me. I arrived in Sydney and discovered white fungal growth in my mouth. I can't fool myself any longer. I couldn't come and pick you up today. I was glued to the toilet. And, while you had your juice, I went into the toilet and threw up mine. When we were having lunch, I hurried off because I almost shat myself. This is it.' His voice trembles. His shoulders hunch further, his fists dig deeper into his pockets. He stares at his shadow and walks faster.

AIDS. The acronym has smeared itself over me, numbing my brain. Like a sinking swimmer, I struggle to thrash my way to the surface and stave off the panic of drowning.

'Do I dare disturb the universe again?'

'It was worthwhile last time.'

And then his low voice. 'I think I've got AIDS, Maria.'

It's been said. Something wrenches inside me. Oh, my dear, sweet friend. What do I do now? How do I take this away from you? I look up and notice strollers gazing at us. I realise I am frowning and my mouth is twisted.

Oh God, no, I pray silently. I swallow the rising lump in my throat. With one hand, I hold my jacket closed in front of me as I feel a cold wind whip at me. I slide my other arm through Jon's and hold his forearm firmly. I can make this worse for him. I can make it better. I have to find resources in me that I've never called upon before. To help him, I must keep control. 'You only think. You don't know.' I sound calm.

'I've done enough reading and self-observation. Remember, I'm a biologist.'

'But you don't know for sure. It could be anything else! You're not a doctor.'

'I've been deceiving myself that it's stress or a nice, normal virus. I have to face it. I'll go for a test when I get back to Adelaide.'

'I'll go with you.'

He stops and hugs me, burying his face in my shoulder and hair. 'I'm so glad you said that. Because I don't know what I'm going to do. You know, we've never really talked about AIDS. It's as if we, somehow, knew we'd be talking about it more than enough one day.'

I feel useless. I don't know where to begin to do something useful. My words sound hollow. 'I'll do what I can. I don't hold stupid prejudices. You should know that.' We resume our walk. 'But I can't believe it.'

'I'm sure it is,' he says and raises his right hand, staring at his trembling palm. 'My life slowly winding down. Losing everything a bit at a time. My homes, my dreams, my love, my health, my life.'

8

ONE DAY, as the spring of 1985 was warming to summer, Jon and I sat talking on my front verandah. Pausing, he took my hands and stared intently into my palms. He murmured several times, and congratulated me on a wonderful life ahead. Hesitantly, he explained he could read palms, although he didn't particularly like advertising it. Knowing your friends' futures was not as illuminating as you might think.

'How do you read palms?'

'It's not so much the palm of the hand, just a concentration on the spirit, and I see things about that person that make sense.'

From that day, he'd often take my hands and read. He

made an impact on my life, giving subtle direction, placing possibilities in my mind that I could pursue or avoid. 'I keep an open mind about these things,' I told him. 'Who knows what else there is besides what we see around us? But it could be autosuggestion, couldn't it?'

'You still have control to a certain extent. This is what is destined for you if you let things be, but you can consciously modify your life, for better or worse.'

'So what do you see?'

'You have pushed yourself, intellectually, beyond what was meant for you, and you'll continue to do so. You'll always have one happy marriage. You're lucky,' he said, looking at me intently. 'And in other ways, you make your luck by being in control of what happens to you and what you do. Rob provides the perfect marital environment for you to be yourself and broaden your horizons. You know you'd be a fool if you gave away such a gem of a man despite the temptations.'

'Sounds great so far. I hope you're right. But will I ever have any kids? I can't see myself as a mum.'

'Yes, you'll have children. And unbelievable as it may seem, you'll make a great mother, but not in the traditional way. Your self, your ambitions, your relationships with Rob and others are too important to you to submerge for the sake of children. You'll have much to teach about what mothering really means, and your children will shine. Rob will be an excellent father, loving and gentle.'

'Shit! You're making my head swim. But I intend to keep two feet on the ground, thank you.'

'That's one of your successful strategies.'

'How many ankle-biters?'

'I definitely see one. And it looks like another, but one will have a greater impact on your life than the other. It'll be special in some way. Don't get me wrong. You'll love the other, but there's something about one of them.'

'What am I going to do with myself for the rest of my days?'

'Lots. I see you picking up the pace, doing more and more. By the time you're in your mid-thirties, you'll be quite well-known. You'll be teaching in some capacity for a long time, but you'll develop another area that you've no idea about now. One that's always been there, just waiting.'

'Hollywood, here I come!' I said, ruffling my hair, pouting my lips, and laughing.

'I don't think you'll be a titillating starlet, darling, but you'll be doing something that others'll know about. I think your achievements will be more valuable than posing naked in movies.' Jon paused and, although he smiled, his face was flushed. He looked seriously into my eyes. 'Your whole life is charmed.'

'It all sounds so unreal, and scary, and exciting. But does that mean that nothing will ever go wrong? There must be rotten times?'

'There are in everyone's life, but the way one deals with them will make them chaotic disasters, insignificant, or turning points. You have the knack of minimising threats before they become disasters. There's no way I can prevent the death of those you love. But you'll be strong and go on. I wish I could prevent your death. The world needs people like you. Your death is here.' He put a still forefinger at the junction of my wrist and palm, a little below my thumb.

I'd never really stopped to contemplate death. As if, by overlooking death, it would overlook me and the ones I loved.

'You'll have a long life, well into your eighties. Happy and healthy. To the end, your mind'll be pumping out lucid thoughts and theories. And then, you'll just die. You won't know you're dying, and that's the best way.' I tried to visualise myself old, an eighty-year-old woman, thinking and feeling as I did now, my self caught in a slowing body that limited my physical span but not my mental expanse.

'I'm scared of death, Jon. I've never faced it. I've never really faced anything bad in my life. I've got no idea how I'll react.'

'Well, there are crises in your life. You'll get through and you'll be getting on with things after them. When you're about twenty-seven, twenty-eight, you'll go through some sort of crisis or turning point, some sort of death.'

'Oh God! We intend to have a baby about then. Or is it one of my parents? We're talking about events only two or three years away.'

'I don't know. I don't think so.' Jon frowned, staring into my palms, heat rising in his face. 'I can't really tell, but it involves a death. After that, you know, things'll get better.'

'Another crisis?'

'Very late fifties. Early sixties. I think it's another death. But you'll go on. One of your children will be very close and will remain a great support until you die.'

'Rob?'

Jon nodded slowly. 'I think so. He'll die quite a few years before you.'

I felt a dead weight explode in my heart and hurtle into my stomach. I had always known, deep inside, I would lose my life's love, and have to continue without him. I had tried to visualise it but, at the point of his death, my visions ended. 'Oh no,' I say. 'I won't be able to face it. I'll die too.'

Jon stroked my palm. 'You'll be okay. You'll continue to make something special of your life for that's what Rob will have always encouraged you to do. And he'll be there somewhere helping you. I'll be there too.'

I tried not to think about it. That evening, Rob had his palm read while I listened feverishly. Jon held his gentle paw. 'You'll be a successful man, a happy man whose life is full of love. You'll have big career decisions in your mid thirties. You'll make a great father.' Jon paused. 'And you'll probably die in your early sixties.'

That night, Rob and I hugged in bed. 'Death frightens me too,' Rob whispered, nuzzling close to my ear. 'We'll have to make the most of our time together.'

The next day, on the same front verandah, I was studying my

hands while Jon looked on. 'What about your life?' I asked him. Jon looked away, clenching his hands into fists. 'Let me have a look.' I grabbed his hands, uncurled the fingers, and made ignorant attempts to 'read' them. 'Well, you've got a lifeline and a heartline and lots of little lines.' I laughed.

Jon did not laugh. His face was severe. 'I try to avoid looking at my hands because their messages get in the way of my hopes and plans.' He faced me, hands open with palm upwards. 'But at least I won't get old and ugly. I dread old age with its humiliations, and it looks like my vanity and wrinkle cream are quite unnecessary.'

'When?'

'You're going to know everything, aren't you?' The fore-finger that had traced the years and years of my life and had pointed to the death of my partner, now found a junction in his own palm. I wondered how he felt with his finger resting on the end of his life.

'My death will be painful. You see, I won't want to die, but I'll know for a long time that I'll be dying. I don't know why I'll die. It's here, but I don't understand it. But that's not really the important thing. What is really difficult is knowing that all I have will be slowly and deliberately taken away from me. When I die, I'll have nothing left.

'See how my life is split in two, here on my hand? See the many criss-crosses, confusing junctions and frustrating dead-ends? That's how it's been, and here is how it will be. More of the same. More dead-ends until the ultimate dead-end – '

'If it's true, and I hope you make mistakes, you'll have something when you die. Not much maybe. Not significant enough to be printed in your hand. You'll have me.'

He leaned his head on my shoulder. 'But you're terrified of death.'

'Yeah, well, I'll have to introduce myself sooner or later. But let's not hold our breath waiting for the day, hey?'

Jon raised his head and smiled. 'As I said, I try to control it, modify my destiny. I've got things I want to do. Like raise a child, and that's long-term. So I won't give in to the reaper that easily.'

'According to that,' and I pointed to his palm, 'how much time?'

'I won't live to see much of my thirties.'

I close my hand over his palm. The trembling ceases. My arm instinctively circles his waist. Such a thin man. How this must be eating away at him. These fears have been haunting him for months, and he's faced them alone.

'Don't say anything to Kevin. I want to know for sure first. I need time to work it out. No one in Sydney is to know. Let's enjoy the next few days. We might never get this opportunity again.'

'I never did like Sydney, Jon.'

We begin our walk back.

We go to restaurants, dancing, shopping; see old friends who reminisce about college days and Jon's cheeky taste for fun. We chat and smile. Now and again, we exchange pained looks.

Kevin shows us his cosy room in the nurses' home, introduces us to his favourite gay clubs and pubs and bookshops in Oxford Street. Jon watches Kevin, absorbs his words, his gestures, laughs at appropriate moments, asks appropriate questions. He reaches out to touch his arm gently.

We sit in a Mexican restaurant and raise glasses for a toast. I realise Kevin isn't wearing his gold ring and that for the first time I cannot drink more than half a glass of champagne without feeling nauseated.

Jon and I walk along beaches and cliffs. Each landmark evokes a reminiscence and a reflection on what had been and what is to come.

We buy some pieces of pottery at the Rocks, and as we trudge along the streets, we talk of heritage and change.

At the top of the Centrepoint Tower, we look down on the people. And we laugh hysterically as we both dash away from the window, and cling to the rail near the lift. We both feel like we're going to throw up. 'Imagine how they'd put up a guard rail and a sign saying, "Danger! AIDS-infected chuck!" I know what's making me giddy. But what's wrong with you?'

'Maybe I've got sympathetic nausea, worrying about you.' We hug each other, trying to stifle our laughter.

'Phantom AIDS!'

Out at the Heads, we sober up at the thought of countless suicides that have been contemplated. We watch the waves pound the shore and shiny speedboats full of tanned, care-free people who don't appear to understand what winter is.

On a flat rock overlooking the Bridge and the open span of water, we lie down and feel the warm stone against our backs, the rays of sunlight warming us from a serene blue sky above. The chill in us isn't thawing.

'You know at the Centrepoint,' Jon begins, his arms behind his head, his eyes shut tightly, 'you seemed to feel sick. Could it be psychosomatic? I mean, knowing I've got AIDS – '

'You might have AIDS,' I interrupt.

'Well, could you be worrying about catching it yourself? I mean, you might not know all the facts about it.'

I lean on one elbow and look at him. I poke him in the abdomen, making him sit up with a gasp. I tickle him under the arms until he begs me to stop or we'll both fall into the water below us. I grab his face in my hands and kiss his mouth. 'Don't you dare think that again or I'll become very violent.'

'I believe you would too, you hot-blooded Mafia queen!' He tugs at my hair.

'What kind of queen are you, hey?'

We hold each other tight.

We take daily strolls down Oxford Street. I am drawn to the street for, despite the usual commercial pretences, there is a refreshing openness and humour about the shopkeepers and the customers.

'He's got it,' Jon says, pointing out feeble-looking, troubled-looking men. He discusses the marks on their faces, the thin angular bodies attempting dignified walks.

The night before we leave, we stay at Gary and Linda's, old friends of Jon's, a warm and hospitable couple. Kevin stays too. We're not a happy threesome. Going to collect an over-night bag for Kevin in the nurses' home we found the car had been broken into. Jon's leather jacket was gone, and Rob's camera, the one I'd given him for his twenty-first. 'That jacket's been all over the world with me,' Jon muttered bitterly.

'I've always hated this city!' I yelled into the empty street.

So we go to sleep in poor spirits, Jon and Kevin on a mattress in the lounge, and me in the spare room. I lie awake, listening to my own anger and the whispers from the lounge-room.

In the morning, we pull up near a train-station on a busy street. Kevin kisses me before he gets out. 'Take care of this kid,' he says cheerily, but the firm pressure on my arm belies his nonchalance.

He gets out. Jon does too. I can see their two slim male frames close together. One moves away a little. The other follows. I cannot hear them. I see Jon's hand squeeze Kevin's momentarily, down by their sides. I see Kevin's fingers disentangle themselves. He takes a quick step back-ward, turns, and jogs away.

Jon stands still, hands in his pockets, until Kevin is lost in the crowd.

He turns, sits hurriedly in the car, and slams the door. He grips the steering-wheel, white knuckles, whiter than his face. He squints into the rear-vision mirror as the car roars into life, his foot pressing heavily on the accelerator. His eyes are ringed with lines of strain. I think he's about to break down, get out of the car, and run after Kevin.

But he doesn't. He looks at the road ahead, sighs, and

smiles. The car moves slowly forward.

I sit silently, looking out my side window so Jon doesn't see my eyes.

Jon reaches out and clasps my leg. 'It's okay. I'm a survivor, you tell me. Let's enjoy this drive.'

'I can't see anything!' I blurt out. 'It's not fair, Jon.'

Jon speaks steadily, staring straight ahead. 'Well, things aren't always fair.' He takes my hand. 'Sometimes you care too much. You have to let it all be. I understand your tears, but I need your practical concern too. To show me logic and exits when I can't find the way out.'

'I'm pretty hopeless at that sort of thing.'

'No. You've been great.'

Soon, the last of Sydney is left behind and the natural beauty of the landscape begins to breathe some peace into us.

The fast red car becomes our shell through which we view the passing scenes. We laugh, bicker lightheartedly, listen to comedy tapes as rain drizzles on the window, and the flat plains appear grey and lifeless. We talk about our childhoods. We talk about AIDS.

We spend the night at a motel in West Wyalong. We read excerpts from a book on AIDS Jon has bought in Oxford Street, familiarising ourselves with the scientific terminology, the symptoms, disorders, naturopathic remedies, legal and medical consequences. We speak about 'it' in clinical, detached terms. I wonder whether there is a book that deals with the emotional, psychological and personal issues.

We eventually get to sleep, in separate beds next to each other. I wake during the night and look across to Jon's sleeping form, dimly lit by the moonlight coming from the window.

I wake again to sounds of water running, and the toilet flushing. Jon is coughing. He shuffles back to bed, and runs a hand over his bottom sheet. He has taken off his t-shirt. He climbs back into bed with a low groan.

I'm sleeping in a room with a person who probably has AIDS. It seems so strange, so scary. When it all comes down to it, this is just my dear friend who may be very sick.

We arrive in Adelaide on Sunday night. It's cold and rainy. As we turn into my driveway, we both sigh with relief. Jon is very tired, his face drawn, but he insists on carrying my suitcase into the hallway. I'm also tired, slightly nauseated, and glad to have ended the driving at fast speeds on empty roads while the rain poured down.

The house is silent. Rob's left for a conference in Canberra. But in the kitchen is a beautiful basket of red and white carnations, and a card welcoming me home. 'It's really different on your own,' it says. 'There's a feeling of something lacking in my life. (I know how you must feel when I go away!) The worst part is that now I have to go away without seeing you. But I'm sure you had a great holiday and you'll have lots to tell when I get back.'

Jon takes the card from my hand and reads it slowly. A pained smile skirts his face. He puts the card on the kitchen bench, and gently touches a white carnation.

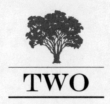

TWO

*The real voyage of discovery consists
not in seeking new landscapes but
in having new eyes.*

Marcel Proust

9

FRIDAY MORNING seems to be asleep, dragging its feet through each minute. We have only been back at school for a fortnight and already I feel as if I need a holiday. I escape at lunchtime after a few explanations to friends.

On the first Monday back at work, Jon and I had been teased for the scandalous liaison we'd made in Sydney. We played along. It made us laugh, the way we always had.

As I drive into town, I hope that tomorrow will restore us to an honest normality – or to the usual dose of dishonesty. By tomorrow my nausea will begin to subside and tomorrow night, Jon and I will dance, grateful for life.

Tomorrow. What is this niggling voice that responds with a quietly crashing 'No'?

At Alfrescos, I sit on a stool near the window waiting for Jon. I don't have my usual interest in passers-by, in groups seated inside the place. I feel nervous. I can only think of two things – how Jon must've been feeling all morning; and how wonderful it'll be to end this day.

On Thursday, Jon didn't come to work. He went for the test. As I dealt with students, papers, bells, I thought of his fear, illness, and humiliation, and my day suddenly seemed so trivial.

As soon as I got home, I rang him. Robbo told me he'd gone for a walk.

I didn't eat very much. My stomach felt bloated. 'Why don't you go and see him?' Rob suggested after dinner. 'Just keep in mind that it's highly unlikely to be AIDS.'

'Reassure me,' I begged, holding his hand.

He kissed mine and held it to his mouth. His moustache and beard tickled my skin. 'It couldn't happen to him.'

'Now I *know* I need to worry.'

Jon sank into his chair. 'Well, I've done it. Now I have to wait till next Friday afternoon.' He looked at the cuckoo clock. 'They asked quite a few questions. Reasons for the suspicion. Enquiries about my way of life. Personal data. Where relevant and necessary, I told the truth. But I gave myself a different name, a different job, a different residence. They assured me of the strictest confidence, and I'm sure they meant it, but what if it leaks out? There goes my respectable existence if they find out I really have a decent, heterosexual virus after all.' He smiled drily.

I offered platitudes and asked questions.

'They were encouraging. They said I'd be able to do something about it, but I get panicky at the thought of next Friday.'

'Remember, I'm coming with you. If you still want me to.'

'I do. I'll need help to stay in control if I'm going to get through.' He looked up to the ceiling, palms open. 'A scourge on Sodom.'

'Don't give in to such thoughts!' I snapped. 'Don't let years of religious indoctrination sneak in through the back door.'

The week wore on. Same routines in the classroom, same conversations in the staff-room. Everything seemed suspended in time. There was Jon, picking over morsels at lunch, ignoring students who wanted to engage in the usual lively debates.

On Thursday, I asked for Friday afternoon off, telling Peter, the deputy principal, I had a doctor's appointment. His eyes were gentle and understanding. I had the feeling he knew I was lying.

Jon is late. Perhaps he won't show. I resolve to sit and wait all afternoon if necessary. What else could I set my mind to?

Forty minutes later, without breakfast or lunch, I'm feeling queasy. I buy a tuna salad roll. The bread tastes dry, the tuna too salty. I leave half of it in its plastic wrapper. These symptoms have plagued me since the holiday in Sydney, I realise.

In fifteen minutes, I see Jon walking down the street, shoulders hunched, hands in pockets, a frown etched into his forehead. He seems to be counting the cracks and stains on the pavement. He sees me and sits down next to me, apologising because he has spent the morning sick in bed. He'd fainted in the shower. Luckily, Robbo was there, heard the thud, and helped him back to bed.

'It must be nerves,' I say.

'It's common for people with AIDS to faint in showers,' he replies.

He sips an orange juice slowly, as if to prolong every precious second. I buy an iced chocolate drink, hoping the milk will soothe my stomach and the sugar my anxiety. We listen to others laughing and arguing over their coffee and gelati. The warm smell of coffee wafts around us, and the occasional hiss of the cappuccino machine urges us to hurry.

'Well, let's go.' Abruptly, he climbs off the stool. I stumble over my bag in my haste to be alongside him.

We walk down Rundle Street, Frome Road, and turn in to North Terrace. Jon seems calm and controlled, discussing the reading he's been doing on ways to slow down the degenerative processes of AIDS. I begin to feel that everything is too commonplace – the people, the shops and buildings – too safe and homely.

Across the road from the Royal Adelaide Hospital is the Sexually Transmitted Diseases Clinic. As we turn to enter the dark glass doors, I glance back. People waiting at the bus stop watch us curiously, grimly.

In the waiting-room, we exchange glances with others.

Jon approaches the counter. 'I'm here to find out the result of an AIDS test,' he says simply. I blanch at his words. It seems dreamlike to be making such a request.

The nurse behind the counter, maintaining her official demeanour, indicates we'll need to go to the other office for, as she puts it, 'your particular results'. She smiles as if she's pleased with her discreet manner, unaware of the ambiguity of her words. 'Particular results'? Is it a special office for HIV tests or HIV positive results?

We walk back along a hallway and go through other glass doors. Inside, the walls are covered with AIDS publicity: racks of booklets and pamphlets are on either side of two lounge suites. 'Must expect a crowd in here,' Jon mutters.

We sit down, avoiding looking at the man on the seat next to us. He is tall, tanned, blonde, well built. His blue faded jeans are torn, his white t-shirt hugs his muscular chest. He looks like a rugged Australian beachcomber but without the arrogant self-awareness characteristic of the species. He stares into the distance, left hand clasping right fist, elbows leaning on his knees, pretending we're not there, perhaps pretending he's not here either.

Jon leafs through a pamphlet on how to prevent being infected by the HIV virus. 'A bit late,' he mutters, and shoves it back into the stand.

Receptionists with smart office heels tap their way to and fro behind the long grey counter, neat and efficient. They have placid smiles, breezy voices as they ask each other for papers and files. They consciously avoid looking across the counter.

A young doctor wearing a white coat comes out of an adjoining room and silently beckons the man next to us. The man rises quickly, rubbing his hands on his back pockets and walks slowly towards the doctor. The door shuts silently behind them.

'I'm next,' Jon says. I touch his arm. My heart is beating faster and louder, my palms are clammy and cold. I wonder how he's feeling.

No, it won't be, I tell myself again. And the ominous voice from inside retorts, 'Yes, it will.' Not to my friend, I insist, not in my commonplace world.

I have no time to hear the response welling up inside me. Another door has opened. A thin young doctor is walking towards us, his white coat billowing around him. His pale blue eyes shine behind his glasses as he beckons us to follow him.

Jon rises first. I follow, deliberately numbing my mind. I will wait now.

We enter a small, windowless office that sends claustrophobic shivers racing through me. The desk takes up the main area and the doctor's chair is squeezed against one wall; the two chairs opposite the desk are prevented from resting against the other wall by a potted palm tree.

We squeeze into our chairs. The yellowish fluorescent light directly above us casts fragile shadows. The palm tree's leafy fingers tickle our necks. Jon's fists are clenched as he struggles to free his neck and shoulders from the plant's clutches.

The doctor leafs through some papers. He places one steadily on his desk. I read Jon's alias at the top, but the doctor's hand deftly conceals most of the rest.

'You came in a week ago, is that right?' he asks. His voice is warm, his gaze behind the shiny glasses level and friendly. I notice his fingers are bony, his complexion pale.

'Yes.' Jon's voice is throaty, deep.

'Yes,' the doctor echoes and glances once more at the paper.

Suddenly he is speaking, with the level gaze and slow, steady voice. I feel my mind has been transported miles away where it must struggle to register what's being said. I want him to slow down so I can take it all in, so I can think beyond the frothing panic, so I can breathe deeply to avoid the sensation of falling.

Control, I scream silently at myself. 'You have tested positive, you have tested positive' whirls round in my mind.

Jon has jerked forward in his chair, his hands visibly trembling, clenched into tight fists on tense knees. His breathing is shallow. He stares at the paper on the desk as if his eyes could burn into it. I can see the muscles in his jaw, the vein in his temple, working frantically.

My arm encircles him, hugging his stiff body to me. My other hand unfolds one tight, wet fist and wraps around his fingers. He squeezes it. I can't see.

'I know this is a blow. Try to relax. It's time to get into the right gear to try and beat it,' the doctor says gently.

Jon nods. 'I'm all right,' he says loudly, forcing his voice to clear, forcing his body to sit back. 'What do I do now?'

'We'll try to organise treatments. For the specific matters like your stomach symptoms, and the fungal growth in your mouth. We may be able to get you AZT, but you understand how expensive it is. Please believe me, AIDS is not an automatic death sentence. If we arrest this, if you watch your health, you can continue to work and live a normal life for many years. You can cut out the crap in your life and fill your time with meaning.

'You mustn't give in to it. Build your inner strength. Out there, you may think you're alone, but you're not, and we'll give you all sorts of advice when you need it.'

The doctor turns to me. 'You may need to make a few arrangements. You may need a test.'

'No, she won't,' Jon says. 'Maria's my closest friend, but there's no sexual intimacy.'

'My apologies. It's rare for a friend to be present at times like these. Jon, you'll need people who'll take care of you, keep you going through the rough times. But you're going to get some benefits out of this. You'll learn how strong you are, what you're capable of, and who your friends are. You'll also learn about prejudice and ignorance, unfortunately.' He smiles at me. 'It looks like you've got yourself a strong friend.'

'What can I do?' I say.

'Be there. Listen, support. Take some of the weight off

Jon's shoulders. Be a target when he needs to vent some anger. I don't think you'll be at a loss.'

The doctor and Jon exchange questions, appointments are made, more information gathered. I admire the doctor's assuredness and Jon's dignity and steadfastness. I vow to be the same.

We rise to leave. It has only been about fifteen minutes. At the door of the office, the doctor pauses and looks at us warmly through his glasses. 'Take it in your stride. There are two hundred and thirty-four people living with HIV that we know of in South Australia. We've only had two deaths. Most of us are surviving very well. We've come to terms with it, made the appropriate changes in our lives. We're going to beat this thing. I know I lead a fuller life now than I ever did. Any little thing I accomplish means so much. I may have less time, but it'll be time well spent. I've actually started to live now that I know I don't want to die.' He removes his glasses and shakes our hands firmly and warmly.

Jon and I walk out of the office of a calm doctor who just happens to be HIV positive. I feel reassured.

I am about to tell Jon this as we reach the stairwell that'll take us down to the road. I'm on the second step when I hear his sobs behind me. Jon is against the wall, face hidden behind trembling fingers. He cries out, and groans shake his body. The passive stance in the doctor's office was what Jon would call typically Anglo-Saxon: be controlled, don't let others see your pain. Even now he's struggling to squash the sobs.

I grab his shoulders and he turns into me; the force of his feelings pushing me into the wall, his head buried in my shoulder. 'Let it out,' I whimper.

We hear footsteps coming up the stairs. With much effort, Jon pulls himself away from me to the other side, frantically wiping his face with his sleeves, steadying his body. 'Let's go,' he whispers hoarsely and begins to go down the stairs just as a forlorn figure of a man comes around the corner, the tension visible in his furtive eyes.

Out on the street, on busy North Terrace, Jon says, 'Let's go to the Botanic Gardens.' We walk, arm in arm. He begins to talk, relentlessly voicing his fear, anger, sense of enveloping helplessness.

I listen and look around me. It is so strange to see people going about their ordinary existences. Why doesn't the world stop, just for a minute, so we can get our moorings? If the result had been different, we'd be heading back to Alfrescos with the same camaraderie and spring in our step as everyone else about us.

The gardens are still: majestic trees with life spans far outdistancing human ones; manicured lawns and thriving plants.

We walk for a while and then sit on a white bench on high ground, looking over the lawns and the meandering paths. Alongside, a tall tree casts shadows around us. The afternoon sun is warm. We sit for two hours on that bench, conscious of the foreboding view of the austere hospital buildings above the tree canopy. I hope my voice doesn't betray my tears. I offer encouragement while Jon talks. I can't believe that, sooner than I'd thought, I'll lose my dear friend. I feel useless.

'It's like a passenger travelling in my body,' Jon says, trying to visualise the AIDS virus. 'When it completes its tour, I'll be a corpse. My body has turned on me.'

He talks of the isolation he feels having a disease that solicits disgust and damnation. He'll have to fight the disease and the fear of it in others. He repeatedly airs the importance of each minute in his life. He has goals, a new set of objectives: to get treatment, to change his diet and to set new attitudes to living. No alcohol, lots of good natural food, plenty of sleep. He'll learn to tolerate the tedious procedures he will need to adopt: to change his bedlinen each day after the nightsweats, to disinfect his home, to take drugs to control the symptoms, to put a chair in the shower, to avoid people with common colds and viruses, to organise his money, fix his insurance, make a will. It's ironic, he says, that although others believe he's a danger to them, their common illnesses could easily kill him.

'It sounds so extreme, but it's so necessary for this extreme disease,' he says. 'If I had leukemia or a respectable cancer, I'd only have to whisper it once and they'd fall at my feet with support and sympathy. If I tell them what I've really got, I'll have to watch them back off. I'm a twentieth-century leper! I can't even tell my parents. How do I tell these two old folks that their son won't be around to bury them?'

'What about Kevin?'

'He'll be free one day. When I'm organised, I'll tell him. I'll show him I intend to be around for a while so he'd better prepare to do some of his nursing on me.'

'He may need a test, Jon.'

He thinks for a bit. 'Yes, I'll tell him. But he won't have it. I know it.'

'What about Robbo?'

'I can't tell him yet. He won't be able to take it and then I won't either.'

A young father with a baby bundled into a knapsack on his back strolls by. Jon sighs. 'You know what's hardest? No more plans of travels. No more thought of adopting a child or resuming a long relationship. I should've had this test years ago. But who ever thought then?'

He rubs his face, and snorts. 'I could just as well castrate myself for that pathetic little appendage is going to be absolutely useless. At least it can't get me into any more trouble.'

He looks up at the sky, squinting at the sun. 'One day, I won't see this. The days before I die must be filled with something. What I'm doing now is what I want to do most. So I'm going to keep teaching and hang on to my independence for dear life. But I also want dignity. Let people believe the lies while I live out my truth. It'll be an achievement to carry on as normal, to function so fully that no one knows or guesses otherwise.'

The sun is sinking. It's getting colder. 'I'm going to do the best I can to live,' Jon decides as he scans the orange sky. 'Really live.' He winds an arm around me and hugs me closer to him. 'Maria, promise me one thing. I'm not a hero or martyr and I know rumours and suspicions will spread as I degenerate. Promise me you'll never say a word about what I've got to anyone at work, or your friends. Rob can know. I'll be speaking to him myself about drugs and treatments. But no one else. I couldn't bear the pity or the humiliation of it all.'

Jon gently rubs a fist on his thigh. 'I can only cope with this disease if I believe everyone sees me as normal. So lie for me, how ever long it takes.'

'Yes. I understand why you want it so, but it hurts me to think it has to be this way.'

'When I'm dead and it doesn't matter anymore, promise me you'll let them know.'

'That'll be years from now. I'll be old and grey and will have to look up addresses.'

Jon shakes his head. 'No, it won't be like that. My palm, remember?' He holds it out in the setting sun and traces his lifeline with a forefinger.

'You said destiny can be changed.'

'If only I'd known when I was just HIV positive.' He presses at the end of his lifeline and takes my hand and traces mine. With a smile, he looks at me. 'You won't need to write letters. But you can write all this down, and all that's going to happen, and let everyone know.'

'You should write it, Jon! I won't know what to say!'

He stands up and holds out a hand. 'Let's go then.'

We leave the gardens, knowing that somehow the tangle will unravel itself, regardless of our dreams and nightmares. Jon intends to go to the market and buy fresh fruit and vegetables and an assortment of health products. I offer to walk home with him, or drive him. He wants to walk, to get some exercise, and he wants to go alone. 'You can only travel part of the way with me in this,' he says with a warm smile. 'That'll be a helluva journey anyway. I must learn to traverse the rest of the desert on foot and by myself.'

Suddenly, a woman's voice is calling us. She is running down North Terrace to where we stand on the corner of East Terrace. It's Lizzie, Kevin's sister, red curly hair flying, freckles jumping on her animated face. 'Hi! How are ya?' We exchange conversation about work, about Kevin. 'End of the week,' she says. 'You both look a bit tired.'

Jon laughs. 'Yes, I am rather tired. I'll have to have a long sleep one day.'

After Lizzie has gone, we hug each other. 'I was good, wasn't I? She didn't guess a thing,' he says with a chuckle. He kisses me and walks away.

I watch his shuffling, tense-shouldered, fists-in-pockets walk.

My promise will be put to the test at a gathering of work colleagues at Jim's house. I don't really want to go, but I accept that it's part of the promise, part of Jon's need for normality and control.

When Rob and I arrive at Jim's house, he tells us that Jon has rung to say he can't come. Several people exchange good-natured comments about Jon's hectic nightlife. As the evening wears on, I'm told several times that I look tired. 'It's the end of the week,' I explain.

Someone tells a joke about AIDS and people laugh uproariously. I sense my body freezing, and anger bubbles inside me. Rob catches my glare. I steady myself by fixing my eyes on him until the moment has passed. I would've laughed too, before I'd walked with Jon along Manly Beach, and this thought bothers me a great deal.

10

BY THE NEXT FRIDAY, life has decided to bestow two more challenges, stoke the emotions while they're still on fire.

My parents have left for a nine-week holiday in Italy. Life without them around has a certain instability and, coupled with the imbalance of Jon's situation, has left us feeling precarious. We lack a centre. We visit our parents' house, my first home, and the stillness and smell of a closed, empty house is unnerving. As I wander through touching items that stir memories, sitting pensively on their bed where my brother and I romped every Sunday morning, and looking at their photographs, I know this is what it'll be like one day without them. With their death, a stillness will blanket our old home.

I explain my feelings to Jon. 'To think that adults leading such full and independent lives still see their parents as their focus. Even death won't erase that bond,' he reflects.

'Well, death won't erase my bond to you either.'

'I feel that too. You're very lucky. You have great depth of feeling and commitment, but it makes you very vulnerable. What would you do if your parents never returned from their holiday? If they died in Italy?'

'Don't say that! It's the longest time I've ever been separated from them.'

'What would you do?' he persists.

I try to see myself, my parents dead. But I can't contemplate it. 'I don't know, I don't know!'

'It'll come about eventually, and you'll develop resources when you need them,' Jon says quietly.

And Jon's death will come about eventually, and I will have to learn to deal with it too. Nothing can replace the love and understanding of a good parent and nothing the joy of a good friend.

The other challenge has been advancing stealthily for weeks. I still feel nauseated at times, experience bouts of dizziness, and feel my abdomen is bloated. I don't feel like eating, particularly my old favourite Chinese curries. One evening, Rob and I are cooking a Chinese meal while my brother watches on. He is still in his work clothes.

Rob reaches for the curry powder. 'No. No curry.' I stop him.

'You're kidding!' Tony says, and puts a calloused hand on my forehead. 'You must be fucked.' He tousles my fringe. The smell of his overalls sends a new wave of nausea through me. 'You stink,' I say as I shake away his hand with annoyance.

'Jesus, what do you expect? You can't be a fitter and turner in an office!'

On Saturday night, on our way back from Sydney, Jon and I stopped at a Chinese restaurant in a tiny country town. I sat back, having eaten only a third of my combination curry. 'I'm not enjoying this.' I pointed to my plate.

'That's very unusual for you. You're rather masochistic when it comes to hot curries.'

'I feel so bloated, as if I'd swallowed a watermelon.'

Jon laughed, but I drank two glasses of lemonade before I felt any better. I told myself I was worried about Jon, about driving at night on lonely highways, and my irrational subconscious kept harassing me with ridiculous thoughts about the likelihood of catching AIDS in a little car with windows closed against the cold and rain, breathing each other's air.

On Friday, I decide to visit a doctor in case I'm developing another severe stomach virus.

In the waiting-room, I meet Maria and her fiancé. In two months, I'm to be her matron-of-honour. She looks so happy. I try to be bubbly and explain casually I think I'm coming down with something.

She seems to accept what I say. She's concerned about Mike. A lump has appeared on his back and she fears that it's cancer; she's frightened that this love will die too, this time literally.

So much talk of death around me, I silently groan. I reassure her and feel so weird, almost repeating word by word some of the useless platitudes I tell Jon.

The doctor is a practical, gentle character. I launch into an explanation about stomach viruses, nausea and dizziness.

He knows me well and asks how I'm feeling emotionally. Could it be stress? Quietly, I relate to him the events of the last three weeks. He listens and nods in respect and understanding. 'So it definitely could be stress,' he concludes. 'Or pregnancy.'

I chuckle. 'No. I'm off the pill hoping to get pregnant in a few months, but I've only had one period. I couldn't get pregnant that quickly.'

'Why not?' he asks, raising his eyebrows.

'Well, I'm keeping a chart so it's been safe when we've made love. I'd like to get pregnant towards the end of the year.'

'When was your last period?' he asks with a smile.

I calculate mentally. 'Six, seven weeks ago,' I reply slowly.

His eyebrows rise again. 'That's unusual for you.'

'Yes, yes it is. I hadn't thought much about it. Anyway, couldn't emotional stress have played havoc with my system?'

He rises and opens the door to his examination room. 'Come. Let's just check.'

'Oh, I'm sure I'm not pregnant. I've been keeping a chart. I'm positive it's a virus or stress.'

'Let's eliminate this possibility then,' and he walks into the examination room.

'It's a great idea. A good holiday for you. Just be careful. Remember what you thought of Sydney when the two of us went. Just don't disappear into dark corners of discos with tall, dark, handsome strangers.' Rob's green eyes twinkled. We'd been preparing our evening meal while I told him of Jon's plan to go to Sydney for a holiday.

'Depends what they're offering,' I teased. I held up a cucumber before slicing it up.

'You could easily be mistaken for a high-class prostitute. You'd make quite a sum in a week, and if you split the takings with me – ' Rob pretended to make mental calculations as he stirred the soup.

I made a grab for him and soon we were chasing each other around the kitchen. Until the soup boiled over.

'Some people would say I shouldn't go,' I said, returning to my salad.

'Why not?' Rob tasted the soup.

I laughed. 'On a holiday without my husband, to a wild city like Sydney, with male friends, and gay. God knows what immoral dens I could find myself in!'

Rob laughed and kissed me. 'Since when have other people's judgements worried you?'

'Yeah. I'll go because I don't really give a shit what anyone else thinks. But there's more to me wanting to go, Rob. This may be my last chance for a long time to have absolute freedom. If we have a baby, I'll lose some of that for a while.'

'I thought we were going to be parents according to our own rules.'

'I can't explain this sense of urgency. I need to reassure myself that I'm independent and strong. So when I find myself tied to a dependent little baby, I'll know I could once venture out anywhere and I'll remind myself I'll be able to do it again one day. Do you see what I'm saying?'

Rob put his hands around my waist and nuzzled his face into my neck. 'Yeah. So don't get pregnant this year. When you're ready. But honestly, sweetheart, I don't think having a baby is going to make any difference to you. You know what you're like. You know how we intend to raise our child. Having a baby is going to be a forward step for us. It won't take anything away from our lives because we won't let it.'

When we sit down again in his office, he leans back in his chair and gazes at the little indicator. Without looking at me, he asks, 'How would you feel if you were pregnant?'

'Great!' I say. 'A few months early but who cares! It'd be the lift I need at the moment. Although, I'm supposed to be in a wedding in two months and my parents are overseas and I'd like to be strong for Jon. But I knew –' and my voice fades away as he looks at me with a mischievous glint in his eye and a widening smile sparkling on his face.

'Nothing's impossible. As you've found out recently, we must prepare for all sorts of possibilities and, thank God, for you this is a good one.' He hands me the tester. I look at it and it seems ages before its meaning registers.

I cry and laugh simultaneously and wonder how many twists and turns my emotions can be put through. My parents have been waiting for this for so long, but if I tell them over the telephone, they'll worry through the rest of their holiday or cut it short. And how can I be so happy with Jon so sad?

The doctor is resting back in his chair, smiling with delight. I try to voice my inner confusion; this sensation of see-saw emotions; my fear that all I've been through will have had some damaging effect on the little being inside me, Rob's and my child. I tell him I fear a miscarriage.

'Maria, you are a strong young lady. Take it in your stride. Enjoy your pregnancy. Let your friend enjoy being part of it too. I have known many terminally ill people suddenly find a renewed faith, a desire to keep trying to stay alive with the prospect of a birth, a rejuvenation of life.' He shows me to the door. 'Enjoy,' he says.

With the little tester in my hand and my little baby inside me, already spreading a warm glow through my body, I walk to the car. I must go home and tell Rob. Oh God, another phase, another level of existence. I cry my way home, worrying that I might not be able to see the traffic clearly and have an accident, that I'll miscarry and my excitement and anticipation will have been in vain; about the kind of mother I'll be and the effect of it all on Rob.

At home, I wrap the tester in gold paper and tie a delicate white ribbon around it. I wait impatiently for Rob to come home to present him with this gift.

Rob, who is hardly ever late, doesn't turn up. I pace up and down, listening for the familiar sounds of his car, staring out the window trying to recognize headlights in the darkness.

An hour passes. I have made two useless phone calls. Convinced that the possibilities of life and death are beyond my comprehension, I imagine him in a fatal accident, never to see his child. Desperately, I calm myself down and sit in the lounge room.

A few minutes after the hour, Rob arrives. He was in a meeting and was sure he had told me this morning. He rushes to have a shower for we're expected at a dinner dance.

I gaze at the little gift on my desk. I don't want to rush when I tell him. I want it to be romantic, with intimate conversation and reflection. I decide to tell him when we come home and put the tester in the top drawer of my bedside cabinet.

Jon is also at the dinner dance. Determined to live as normally as possible, he doesn't refuse invitations. I keep his secret well hidden. Yet, tonight I want to tell him my secret.

I watch him sit and pick at the rich food in front of him, engaging in sociable conversation. By ten, he's beginning to feel exhausted. 'It's bad for sleep, this AIDS business,' he mumbles bitterly. 'It keeps you staring at your ceiling all night, afraid to close your eyes. You talk to it, condemning it in one voice and denying it in another, and then vowing to kill it. You lie there in the small hours of the morning, waiting for signs. You see your life frame by frame, coloured by fear and regret. Your bed gets cold and your body gets cold and it feels like death, so you get up to make a hot drink and find yourself throwing up in your kitchen sink. You return to bed only to find yourself sweating so much that you have to change your pyjamas. You give yourself pep talks, cite statistics and naturopathic cures, how your white blood cell count has not dropped; how three oranges a morning provide enough Vitamin C to prevent you catching colds.'

Jon looks around to make sure no one else is listening. Friends are chattering, dancing, glancing at us. 'But the most frightening thought you have, which drives you out of bed once and for all is the one where you run through the days, weeks and months of the year and begin to wonder what day will be stamped into history as your deathday.'

Birthday. Deathday. I cannot tell Jon here.

Rob and I are snuggling in bed, hugging each other for warmth. We're talking about Jon and what he'd been saying to me. Throughout the evening, I'd been testing Rob. 'The doctor said I had a bit of a stomach wog. What if he'd said I was pregnant?' Rob had replied just the way I'd hoped. 'Fantastic!' Whenever his hands hugged my stomach, I couldn't resist a warm smile.

So now, I present him with the golden gift. 'I got this today.'

He looks surprised. 'Jewellery! What've you been up to?' He stares at the tester and for the next two hours, before we settle into blissful sleep, we're crying and laughing and feeling as united as two people can ever hope to feel.

11

'YOU NEED TO TELL JON,' Rob says. 'I think he'll want to know.'

It's Saturday night. I need to see Jon. But I don't know whether I'll tell him about my pregnancy.

Jon grabbed my arm and steered me to his desk behind the science laboratories. 'Guess what! I went to a party last night and I met this very interesting woman. Now don't get jealous. You see, we got to talking and she told me how she really wants to have a baby. She wants a man who's willing to put in equal time and co-parent. She's pursuing her acting career at the moment and is headed overseas for about three years. But we've exchanged contact addresses so that when she returns we have this baby.' Jon catches his breath. 'It's perfect. Kevin and I will raise my very own child.'

'Wow! Are you sure she means it?'

'I bloody hope so. I really want to bring up a child, Maria. But I'm gay.'

'Oh, I hope it works out.'

'Well, if it doesn't, I think you'd better get a move on. What's wrong with you? You're Italian, fertile. Why aren't you having kids?'

I made to swipe him with my hand.

'Only joking!'

I knock on Jon's door. Robbo answers and looks pleased to see me. He isn't going out because he thinks Jon might need company.

Jon looks pale. He's keeping a mental record of good days and bad days and today's been a bad one. He'd fainted after a bout of diarrhoea in the morning, had slept most of the afternoon, and could not stomach any meals with meat in them. He had thrown up dinner only minutes before. 'But I've had plenty of orange juice – Vitamin C – to ward off cold and flu nasties. Pity it doesn't kill the big nasty.' He looks over at Robbo. 'This guy's been hovering about me all day, and he's still here. He should be out gallivanting.'

When Jon goes to the toilet 'for the hundredth fart attack today', Robbo and I exchange silent looks. Although quiet and shy, Robbo's reserved manner has always concealed great intensity of feeling. 'He smokes so much,' Jon had often told me. 'I tell him to stay off the dope. He's losing all his money that way, and cigarettes become little ash-heaps in no time. He's too nervous.'

Robbo shakily lights a cigarette and initiates the conversation, something he's never done before. 'He's had a rough day. I got him to bed and he slept, but it's hard getting him to eat. I've got to get him to try.'

Jon comes back into the room. He looks from Robbo to me. 'Would you like me to leave again?' he asks cheekily.

We grin. 'Robbo says you need to eat.'

'Why shove it down my throat when it rushes through my system and out the other end?' He sighs. 'Oh, look, I'm sorry. Yeah, I need to eat. Don't worry, I will.'

'I'll try blander recipes,' Robbo says.

'I'll eat more if you smoke less. I think you've inhaled more nicotine this last week than in your entire lifetime!' Robbo smiles and blows smoke in Jon's direction. Jon pretends to cough. 'I could get cancer from this passive smoking. God! Can you imagine an AIDS infected queen dying of lung cancer? That'll be a first.'

We laugh. Jon turns to me. 'You're not out on the town.'

'Nope. Prefer to be with you. You're a rage anyway.' I realise now is the time to tell him. 'I've got a secret to tell you.'

'I hope it's good. I've had a gutful of bad secrets.'

I nod. I sigh and say very quickly, 'Believe it or not, I'm pregnant.'

I will never forget the sudden shine in his eyes, the delight in his exclamation, the caressing movements of his hands on my arm. His beautiful response makes me cry. I bury my face in his shoulder. 'Mama Maria!' he shouts and tears redden his eyes.

As Robbo adds his congratulations, I see the joy in Jon's face gradually change into a sad wistfulness. 'Hey, Uncle Jon,' I say, 'you should be happier than that.'

'Uncle Jon,' he repeats.

I hold his hand and we sit in silence.

Robbo clears his throat and leaves the room. I don't see him again that evening. Jon's eyes follow him. 'He gets very upset over me. I never thought he'd be able to handle all this, but he's making such an effort. I sometimes hear him crying at night while he smokes on that stuff. Probably what he's gone to do now. A lot of his life is centred around me and that's disastrous. He's given up his idea of going to Sydney to study nursing, but I'm going to insist on it soon. Once I find some new tenants.'

Sternly, he continues, 'You have to be really strong now.' He gently prods my abdomen. 'Keep relaxed and contented. If I see you unhappy or fussing over me, I'll feel horrible. Don't burden me with that. I'm going to have fun watching you get fat and bulbous! I'll push myself to share as much of this birth and child as I can.'

'You've taught me a lot, Jon. I want you to be there to teach my child.'

'I want to be there too, to have an emotional rather than just a biological bond with a child. But whatever happens, you can teach. You know it all although you think you don't.'

He sips water. 'This holds down feelings of nausea. I must organize AZT treatment or at least nausea tablets. But let's talk about other things. Tell me how you found out, how you told Rob, what you intend to do.'

So we talk and laugh and I tell him my joys and fears.

Jon's eyes light up. 'I have a very interesting photo to show you.' He gets up, rummages in a kitchen drawer, and returns. 'Look at this!'

It is a photograph he took of me when we were in Sydney. I had been lying on my back on a rock overlooking the

Harbour. Suddenly, an urge to bare my abdomen to the wintry sun had swept over me. I'd lifted my jumper and tugged down my skirt, but I hadn't been able to explain why to Jon who sat watching with an amused smile. Jon had taken the photo. 'There's something about this,' he'd said at the time.

Now we held the photo in our hands, as if the camera had captured some mystical moment.

'Your baby was with us in Sydney.'

We sit in silence.

'Apart from having this baby, what are you going to do next year?'

'I don't know. Haven't thought about it yet.'

'You and your baby at home all day, and nothing in your mind except shitty nappies, posseting and burping. That's horrendous.'

'Thanks a lot!'

He frowns at me.

'Okay, okay, it's true,' I concede.

'So here's your chance to get out of the routines you've established and make the most of your time before you go back to work.' He pauses. 'Sounds like my situation.'

'Maybe I'll study. I've always wanted to do more.'

'Yes, but study something that will develop parts of you that are dormant. Write, read, think. This could be the start of a new facet of you.'

'I'll organise something.'

'You're very capable. I know from that hand. There's more in store for you and quite a name to make for yourself. Maybe you've already started. Explore yourself. Your background. Your feminism. The things you believe in and constantly nag about. Make a few powerful statements.'

At two in the morning, I decide it's time to go. We've talked for hours and Jon looks very tired. It's coldly crisp outside. Before I get into my car, I say, 'Now promise me you won't tell anyone.'

We hug. Jon places a finger over his lips and whispers,

'My secret of death. Your secret of birth. I'm going to make sure your secret's revealed with a bouncing bundle before my secret ever gets out. After all, that tiny creature of yours just may be worth staying alive for.' He gives my abdomen a final parting touch.

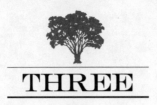

THREE

The troubles of our proud and angry dust
Are from eternity, and shall not fail.
Bear them we can, and if we can we must.
Shoulder the sky, my lad, and drink your ale.

A. E. Housman

12

THE AUGUST DAYS continue to unwind slowly. Each overflows with fears and reliefs, sadnesses and joys. At work, I'm the energetic person my colleagues have always known. With friends, I maintain the happy face they expect to see. No one knows about Jon and only Maria knows about my pregnancy. (She had jumped into my lap for joy when I told her.) I want to wait to tell everyone else until I'm three months because I am afraid of miscarrying.

I am more myself with Jon, but I can't completely release my anger at his daily rendezvous with suffering.

'Gay, single male with the disease in its last stages. I'm right at the bottom, in the mud, for availability of AZT. Heterosexual, married and a mother, and it would be forcibly pumped into my bloodstream. I'm a despicable poofter who deserves what he gets.'

How do I tell him of my dream – Uncle Jon taking my child for walks, and later explaining, opening a mind. How do I respond when he says, 'Aren't you lucky? God's taking me away, an ageing queen, and giving you in return a brand new lovable baby.'

How can I express my wonder at the miracle of life when it juxtaposes the inevitability of death? He wants to know how I feel, what I think, as my breasts ache and my abdomen swells. 'Being pregnant is making me learn about myself, about parts of me I'd forgotten. It's giving me a sense of awe at what my body can do.'

Jon nods and snorts. 'Dying does that too. I didn't realise

how bitter and frightened I could be. I'd forgotten the help-less feeling of weeing my pants in the schoolyard, and the humiliation when it trickled on the school bully's foot and he kicked my balls; that awful anticipation waiting for my father to get home and see my bad report. I'd forgotten how precious life is, but now that it's heading out the door, I feel like running ahead and locking it. Death just doesn't shut up, does it? It talks to you all day long.' Then he covers his mouth. 'Oh, Christ, I'm sorry! What were you saying about being pregnant?'

Only at home, with Rob, do I shed all my masks.

The thirteenth of August is my twenty-seventh birthday. I'm sick in bed with fever and flu and lie there, waiting for a miscarriage, resigned to this fate. Away from the active world, physically still, my mind and my heart have time to race, to play games and quiz each other. Why should I be fortunate enough to survive this physical blow to my preg-nancy? If the baby survives, will it be retarded or deformed? I read pregnancy books, consoling myself with one page and distressing myself with another, and try to sleep, but feverish dreams shake me awake. I think and my thoughts convert the gentle beating of my heart to a heavy thud. My body aches and each twinge has me preparing for a miscar-riage. Every time I stumble to the toilet or shower, I check for blood, prepare to activate a rehearsed agenda: phone doctor, Rob, parents, and bid my child goodbye.

Jon rings. I try to sound cheerful. He tries to sound cheerful. We sheepishly admit we're both fighting back tears. He wants to visit me, wish me a happy birthday, ease my anxiety, have a chat. But he'd be putting himself in danger because his immunity is continuing to deteriorate. 'Visiting you could actually kill me. Your flu is more likely to kill me than your baby.'

There's strain behind his laughter, and behind mine. 'I don't want either of you two to go, you painful shits.'

I recover and my pregnancy becomes easy. My entries in

my pregnancy diary record my amazement at how well everything is going and the dread that it may end.

'The year nine camp to the Flinders Ranges is on again,' I tell Rob.

'Your annual September trek to your beloved Flinders Ranges.' Rob smiles. 'What've you decided?'

'I want to go. I'll do the one-day hikes. The beauty and the fresh air will do me good.'

'I thought you'd want to go.'

'I might not be able to go next year, what with a small baby. I know you'd look after it, but what if there are complications?'

'Well, go and enjoy yourself but –'

'I'll be careful not to over-exert myself.'

Rob laughs. 'That'll be a first!' He holds my hand. 'I'm going to take a week's holiday. I'll go with you.'

I begin to protest.

'I won't get in your way. I won't stop you from doing anything, you know that.' Rob cups my abdomen in his gentle paws. 'But I'll be there to cook for you, to carry you when you can't walk the last five kilometres, to massage your legs and back at night, and to cuddle you in our sleeping bag.'

'It sounds irresistible.'

'I'm glad you're going,' Jon says, finishing some photocopying after school. 'Because I'm not.'

'I was hoping you'd go. We could take care of each other.'

'And poor Rob could take care of us both. No, I won't be able to participate the way I always have, and that'll be painful. You know I love the Flinders, so take some in for me.'

'It won't be the same without you.'

'Nothing's the same.' His smile is resigned.

I walk about thirty kilometres a day. Every evening, I check for spotting and listen for any twinge in my body, telling myself I'll take it easier tomorrow. But tomorrow comes, and I feel refreshed, and I want to go again, crossing the Pound, climbing lookouts to scan the world.

At night, around the campfire, as students chat or sing, I sit with my hands in my pockets, glad that Rob is having such a good time with my students and friends, and wishing Jon were here, warming himself by the fire.

Maria and Mike get married, and I perform and enjoy my duties as matron-of-honour. Maria glows in her joy and Mike cries during the tranquil garden ceremony. I find the courage to make a speech about my love and admiration for Maria, and my respect for her gentle but quick-witted husband. We dance feverishly all night: this is Maria's wedding, and it's going to be as fast and dynamic as she is.

She reintroduces me to John, a tall and solid man with steel-blue eyes. He is dressed with exquisite taste in a checked black-and-white jacket. I'd met him on the night of Mike's buck show when Maria and I had spent the evening together reminiscing. Around midnight there was a knock on the door, and there was Mike crying, drunk, supported by John. Maria took one look at her man and in her typically dramatic way reached out and slapped John squarely on the cheek. 'What have you fucking done to him?'

'Actually, I'm the only one sober enough and big enough to carry him home.' He began to laugh. He pointed to the best man leaning against the door giggling. 'He came along to keep an eye on us.' I giggled too, and Maria stood with hands on hips looking at us.

When John helped Mike to the toilet, Maria whispered, 'He's a fantastic guy, isn't he? We all think he's gay but he's not saying. He just throws out the most obvious comments. His friends think he hasn't quite worked it all out yet. He'll let us know when he's ready, but he knows he won't lose their friendships, that's for sure.'

'So has Mike signed the bit in the marriage contract that says he now becomes an honorary Italian and has to do his share of cleaning out the chicken-yard and stomping the grapes?' John stirs Maria at the wedding party.

'You bet,' Maria says.

I laugh and reflect how he reminds me of Jon. He is the other extreme physically, but so close in personality.

I recall an incident Maria had told me about. She was out for lunch with John when they met a friend of hers in Rundle Mall, a young woman who was a nurse at a suburban hospital. When John made a joke about his being gay, the woman had looked at him in some discomfort. As they prepared to part company, John bent to kiss the nurse's hand in farewell. She tried to pull it away, squealing, 'Oh, I don't want to catch AIDS!' John breathed in deeply so he looked even broader. Looking down on the nurse from his impressive height, he said, 'It takes eleven buckets of saliva for that to happen, darling. I don't dare to think about the kinky kisses you're into!' He continued to stare at her, his steel-blue eyes frozen in distaste, until Maria completed her hasty goodbyes.

I stay out late at parties, go dancing, attend concerts. I work efficiently and energetically and set myself little challenges like running up the stairs to the classrooms.

My obstetrician is proud of me. Rob and I cry with relief as the ultra-scan in September reveals a healthy baby, its little legs crossed, its arms swaying. Its organs are in perfect working order.

Jon's white blood cell count is dropping. His bouts of nightsweats and stomach and bowel symptoms are worsening. He needs to try new medications. He is frequently absent from work or arrives late. 'Had to clean up, calm myself down, and get in the car just in time to throw up and start cleaning up all over again,' he tells me wearily. 'If they ask you what's wrong, just say I'm sick.'

I am being asked, but when it happens I grin and talk about a nasty stomach virus and look like I'm not at all concerned.

Despite his physical deterioration, Jon is beginning to show some acceptance. He speaks vividly of life after death and reads books where people have 'crossed to the other side and returned with good news'. He sighs longingly. 'If I could be guaranteed eternal spirituality, I'd chuck this stinking flesh into the nearest freshly dug grave. But there must be something. I've always believed it. If only God would make this parting easier.'

He reminisces about good times. 'I have lived, haven't I? I mean, really actively lived, not just vegetated my way through an earthly existence. I've made a mark on some, perhaps a scar on others, but I'll leave something of me behind, won't I? Can anyone ask for more?'

At other times, he's quite at ease. 'It's all relative, isn't it? A child dying from malnutrition in Africa would give anything to tread in my footsteps. I must seem wealthy and lucky to millions. To others I am the unfortunate one. But what's really destroying me? Huh! Here's the cycle. From Africa, from the exploited Third World, comes a vengeful virus that the western world ignored until it thought it would cave in to it too.'

There are some peaceful moments to counteract the many chaotic hours. For the rest of the year, Jon turns to literature, reading voraciously, seeking consolation and comparison. He reads passages and poems to me, borrows some of my books and earmarks pages he values.

He consumes Emily Dickinson, T. S. Eliot, William Shakespeare. 'They understood. Dickinson knew death, Eliot knew death in life, and Shakespeare knew the storms of living.' He would accost me before we went to dinner or for a walk with 'Listen to this!' and out would pour the lines that fitted his mood.

'Emily Dickinson! What a woman. She knew how death is an entity, full-bodied. Listen.' He fumbles through pages and reads slowly, and the poetry comes alive:

> *'He fumbles at your Soul*
> *As the Players at the Keys*
> *Before they drop full Music on –*
> *He stuns you by degrees – '*

and on he reads with a smile, and the silence around us in his house vibrates.

One day he comes over for a visit, greets me quickly, and rushes directly into the study, hunting for the Collected Works of William Shakespeare. I stand near the door and wait. Pages ripple through his fingers. 'Here. In this obscure play, "Cymbeline", I found this gem that I wear to deflect the fear of social judgement:

> *Fear no more the lightning flash,*
> *Nor the all-dreaded thunder-stone;*
> *Fear not slander, censure rash;*
> *Thou hast finish'd joy and moan:*
> *All lovers young, all lovers must*
> *Consign to thee, and come to dust.'*

There are days when the past haunts him. 'Life. The way I lived. The events and feelings I experienced. My friend Emily says, "The past is such a curious Creature":

> *Unarmed if any meet her*
> *I charge him fly*
> *Her faded Ammunition*
> *Might yet reply.*
> *My memories haunt me.'*

'T. S. Eliot spoke about memories, didn't he?' I comment.

'Ah, he knew me well, that one. Where is it?' He finds a copy and, with new animation in his face, sits on the edge of his chair, leaning towards me. 'He writes as if he could see me. "They will say: 'But how his arms and legs are thin.' " But look at the strength he gives me here.' The pages burst forth and he reads from 'East Coker'. 'This keeps me on my journey and moving forward to find what I want to find.'

At two in the morning, we sip hot chocolate at his house, the music playing softly. We've been out with friends and now he's exhausted, but the fear of going to bed and not being able to sleep and waking to another day of the same makes him want to sit and talk. His eyes shine. 'I've learned a new poem,' he says with some embarrassment. 'A sonnet. I'm memorising things. I've got to make sure I'm not losing my mental faculties,' and he takes my hands.

> *'When in disgrace with fortune and men's eyes*
> *I all alone beweep my outcast state,*
> *And trouble deaf heaven with my bootless cries,*
> *And look upon myself and curse my fate,'*

and so he continues:

> *'Happy I think on thee, – and then my state,*
> *Like to the lark at break of day arising.'*

13

IN OCTOBER, my parents return from overseas. We told them over the telephone a week earlier that I was pregnant.

My father's hands gently roam over my abdomen. He places an ear to my navel, listening for sounds. He wants to know minutely what is happening to me. He looks at the pictures in my books. 'I couldn't read English when your mother was pregnant. The doctors thought I was too dumb to be told anything. So I want to learn now.'

My mother fusses over my health. I'm not eating enough. I'm not putting on enough weight. She had expected to see me looking far more robust. We laugh as she finds her old knitting needles from a dusty cupboard and begins to make blankets. She begins to plan the end of her employment and looks forward to taking up childcare when I return to work. We tease her. Does she remember what to do? After all, she'd never been a full-time mother with us. How would she handle it? 'I'm ready now. But you're not. If you don't get back to work, after all your study, I'll be greatly disappointed in you,' she says.

'Aren't mothers supposed to want their daughters to do the motherly thing?' Rob asks her with a laugh.

'I was just as good as any of the women who stayed home. Sometimes I think I was better. I was happier and I didn't have to put up with her and Tony all day. So I enjoyed my children. Do you think this wild wife of yours could ever imprison herself in a house with a baby all day long?'

The first two weeks of October are term holidays, and Jon goes to Sydney to tell Kevin and has written to his sister in Africa. She'll meet him in Sydney and together they'll go to Tasmania to see his parents. 'I can do it now,' he says. 'I'm ready to face the consequences.'

I'm ready to let people know I'm pregnant. I have made definite plans for the next two years: I will study, explore my Italo-Australian background and feminist beliefs and return to full-time work in 1989.

Jon is thrilled. 'This is just the beginning.'

Jon rings me twice during the holidays, the first after he's told Kevin. 'I would've hurt him less if I'd hit him with a sledgehammer. He's very worried about me and feels sort of responsible. You know how the doctors say AIDS moves into its final stages if your stress levels are high and your emotions are low. He's had a test. We're waiting for the results, but I don't think he's got anything to worry about. He's being very practical, giving me all the official advice that is passed on to AIDS victims at St Vincent's. But he won't let me use that word. I'm a person living with AIDS, not a victim.'

'I'm glad you've told him.'

I hear Jon's breathing, deep and heavy. 'Kevin's got it all together. I'm just the old fart in the corner who needs bland food and gets exhausted after long conversations. Not that we talk for long. He and his friends are often too stoned to hold a decent conversation.'

'Exaggerating slightly?'

'Yes, I guess so. At their gatherings, everyone rages around me and it's bloody obvious what's wrong with me. So I go to bed and Kevin tells me in the morning that I'd better stop whingeing about feeling isolated when I'm isolating myself.'

'You could try and join in more. The way you do here.'

Jon sighs. 'I'm depressed here. I want to come home where at least I don't have to see a large part of the reason for my depression floating around. I can faint and shit my pants inside my own four walls.'

'Come and live with us.'

'No. I can't burden a pregnant woman.'

'For heaven's sake!'

'Robbo arrived a couple of days ago.' Jon interrupts my protest. 'I think I've convinced him to stay here.'

'Do you really want to live alone?'

'Actually, I ran into my ex-fiancée. She and her boyfriend are thinking of moving to Adelaide. She seems to understand. I've invited them to move in with me.'

'That's good. I can't wait to see you.'

'It's only been a week, but a week is so much time now. I've lost more weight and I've fainted nearly every morning. But I feel better now that I've told Kevin, although seeing him has made me feel nostalgic. If only I could ride back into the past on that laughter.' He seems to choke at the end.

'Hurry home,' I say quietly.

'As soon as I can say goodbye to Kevin. He says he'll do whatever he can for me. He's called me the most wonderful friend he's ever known. Friend!'

'I can imagine how you feel. But try to remember you wouldn't be feeling like this if you weren't sick. You would've accepted the way relationships form and fall apart.'

Jon promises to try. He'll ring me after he's spoken to his parents.

A week later, before preparing to fly back to Adelaide, he does phone. He sounds weary. 'At least Kevin's found out he hasn't got it. But my parents have exhausted me. My sister tried. Facts, data, truth. They don't want to know too much. They detach themselves as if the disease will go away if they don't pay too much attention to it. They're praying for my salvation, but I tell them that I know God, and God knows me. My parents weep and really do care. They just don't know how to convey the love they really feel in a way that'll make us closer together in this. I love them too. But that makes it worse. I'll be glad to get home.'

The final term for the year begins. I am amazed at the amount of attention and support I receive because of my pregnancy. Meanwhile, Jon suffers alone with little support or encouragement, and his frequent absences, even in the first two weeks back, are questioned. What is the 'underlying problem', his colleagues ask. He tells the administration his doctor is finding out.

The following Saturday night, Jon and I discuss our next move. Robbo has collected his things and moved to Sydney. He almost didn't leave. Jon shouted at him in exasperation, holding the door open for him, begging him to straighten out his life. Jon's ex-fiancée will be moving in during the week.

Jon decides to tell the people at work that he has cancer – lymphoma. 'They're getting suspicious. I can't deny there's something seriously wrong. But I want guarantees of support and normality. The symptoms of lymphoma are very similar to those of AIDS, but the reactions it elicits are different. Tell admin about the Friday afternoon when you came with me for the results, but tell them it's cancer. When I arrive later on Monday, I'll tell them too. In that way, it all sounds so marvellously genuine.'

Monday morning is cold and damp. I drive to work rehearsing my monologue, trying out facial expressions in the rear-view mirror. My heart thumps as I approach Peter.

He listens with the same concern he's always shown. I try to look into his eyes so it sounds sincere, but my voice wavers, and I stumble over words. I feel I should shake my head and start again with the truth, but I can't.

In a toilet cubicle, I lean against the door and calm myself. I have shed one skin and superimposed another, which gets further airing as I replay my act to the principal. I have lied to my boss, I tell myself, as I walk out of his office a few minutes later. I am lying to everyone. At least Jon can now get consideration, receive time off, and I can openly show my concern for him. I can drop that mask.

Suddenly, there are interminable questions for which I must invent responses. Is Jon on chemotherapy? Why not? When will he start? What drugs is he taking? Why doesn't he try radiotherapy? How long has he had it? How do you feel about it? How do his parents feel? How long has he to live? A few, those who have heard or seen more mention AIDS. I look at them directly and ask what makes them think it should be that? What are they trying to say? The comments are retracted.

What do they think when I give such vague, stilted replies, eagerly changing the conversation to lighthearted subjects, especially with those I know would support Jon if they knew the truth. How callous they must think I am, a supposedly dear friend who has no idea what is really happening and prefers to talk about her pregnancy, her students' humorous antics, and the latest movies and songs.

One afternoon, I feel more frustrated about the stories than usual. The night before, I'd denied that Jon had AIDS to Maria. Her eyes had followed me, knowing I wouldn't say more. My family members were concerned about Jon. AIDS had been mentioned. All day long, I'd been asked niggling questions by colleagues.

'I hate it!' I tell Jon. 'They must think I'm fickle. They should be made to face the truth and then I could deal with any hypocrisies. I hate all this lying.'

'Oh, that's so important!' Jon says. 'I'm sorry you're so frustrated, you poor thing. What must people be thinking of you!' Before he turns away, he says, 'Don't you think that's a bloody selfish attitude? Just remember who's really in the shit here.' He rushes away.

I stand alone, wanting to cry at my insensitivity. Should I run after him? I gather my books and drive home, grateful that it's the end of the day. We've never fallen out like this and my callousness appals me.

As soon as I've explained it all to Rob, I get in the car and drive over. Jon opens his door and, for a second, we gaze forlornly at each other. Then, we are in each other's arms, crying apologies.

'I won't desert you,' I say before I leave. 'If I lose you as a friend, I've lost something very precious.'

'That's why I panicked. I feel the same. If you abandon me – and when you lashed out, I was terrified that's what you wanted to do – I'll be lost too.' He strokes my hand. 'I just can't let them know. I can't handle all that. Hey, you tempestuous Italian woman, you'll have your moment of truth one day, and then you can fight on for me as much as you want.'

'I'll do just that. I won't care what anyone thinks. I know why I do things and why I think the way I do. You've given me that confidence. I'll toe the line for you now but afterwards, no line, okay? I'll walk where I want to.'

He nods and smiles. 'I know.'

14

IT'S NOVEMBER, and I continue to bloom while Jon is deteriorating. I grow rounder and Jon becomes thinner.

At every visit to my obstetrician I hear the heartbeat, steady and solid. The baby's putting on the right amount of weight. I'm told to watch what I eat, to go easy on rich Italian food.

'I've never eaten more healthily in my life!' I tell Jon as I relate the latest developments.

'Neither have I,' he says with a dry snicker. He puts a hand on my abdomen. 'Amazing what birthing and dying does.'

Jon is seeing death take up residence alongside him, casting a shadow on his daily life. His limbs are becoming thinner, his fingers gaunt and feeble, always cold. He clutches chalk and pens tightly as if a loosening of the grip will prevent him from picking them up again.

One evening, he puts my hand on his heart. It seems light and rapid, fluttering. 'I'm haunted by this sound inside me. To think that one day it'll stop and there'll be silence. When you put your hand here you won't feel this, and you'll know I'm no longer in this body.'

I bite the inside of my lower lip. He senses my anguish. 'Let me speak. I'll come to terms with it if I can talk about it.'

He reaches out his hand to my swollen abdomen. 'You have life inside you too. But one day that life will be in your arms, and the silence inside you will be a happy one.'

A few days later, he receives a call from a sister. His father has had a heart attack. He'll recover but will need to avoid emotional stress. Jon's mother thinks her husband has been agonising over his son. Jon thrashes about with guilt for a few days before pushing it to one side. 'My heart'll give up long before his,' he says.

Jon becomes obsessed with maintaining an organised,

hygienic existence. He worries about the easygoing habits of his tenants. 'They're filthy,' he says with frustration. 'They leave garbage, dirty plates, dirty clothes, mouldy food everywhere. The bathroom stinks. The house hits me with its germs. I sound like a hypochondriac, I know, but I must protect myself because my immunity keeps falling. I clean up after them all the time and I'm so tired after a day at work. They have a cat, a skinny vicious thing that has scratched me twice already. Its litter box sits in the kitchen next to the fridge, and it stinks for days.'

One evening, I visit his place when the others aren't there. I can see the reasons for his frustration, but it's not as bad as the picture Jon has painted. 'I should've known,' he mutters as we try and tidy the kitchen. 'They're London squatters, used to filthy warehouses. When they choke in their own muck, they migrate to an empty site. They say they care about me, and I'm sure they do, but no matter how I try to explain I need cleanliness, they don't understand.'

He scrubs and scours as if he's scrubbing and scouring away the virus itself.

His paranoia concerns me for his system doesn't need this added anxiety. 'Move in with us, Jon. We're not entirely spotless housekeepers, but we'll do the best we can.'

'Maybe. I'll see. But you're pregnant and – '

'Being pregnant doesn't make me an invalid. Look how healthy I am.'

'I can see how healthy you are.'

'Oh, shit. I'm sorry. Words just don't – '

Jon blows some soap suds at me. 'It's okay. You may be healthy, but you're beginning to look like you're developing the most atrocious beer-gut.'

By the end of the month, his immunity level is dangerously low and he's ill in bed for a week. His liver and kidneys are also beginning to fail under the impact of several days of drugs that deal with the symptoms. But no AZT. None is available for him.

He forces himself to get better and, on the following Monday, races to me in the schoolyard. Pale and frightened, he mutters, 'I must talk to you.'

We sit in an empty office. He twists his fingers, his upper body nervously swaying. The shadows under his eyes have become perfect semi-circles. 'Apparently, my immunity is so low, I should be dead. So the doctor said.' A grimace distorts his mouth.

'Well, you're not. You're beating the hearsay and vague medical knowledge. You're willing yourself to live, like you said you would.'

'Yes, I guess I'm succeeding,' but he doesn't look very happy. 'I have felt for some time now, especially during that bout last week, that only my mental and spiritual self was keeping my body going. I have an eerie feeling that my body wants to surrender, but the inner me refuses to evacuate the dying shell.'

'You're a survivor.'

He looks at me sadly. 'I was knocked out last week by a new virus. I'm on medication for it now and it looks like I've almost beaten it.' He looks away momentarily and then turns back, eyes full. 'It's CMV.'

'What's that?' I sense something horrible is descending.

'Cytomegalovirus.'

'Not registering, Jon.' He searches my face.

'I've heard of it, but I don't know much about it.' I begin to feel nervous.

'It's a virus that can be spread through cat litter. I can thank my loving caretakers and their miserable mongrel.'

'Jon, you don't know whether it came from that cat.'

He passes thin fingers through thinning hair. 'It can result in foetal deformities if a pregnant woman comes into contact with it. Maria, you need a blood test. The chances of you having it are minimal. But it does spread easily.'

I don't know what to say. My fear swells into anger towards him.

Jon reaches forward to me, crushing my clenched hands

with his own. 'Oh Maria, I would kill myself now if I knew I could guarantee you didn't have this. I can't bear doing this to you. Oh God, I'm so sorry!' He weeps silently.

My body shivers, and my heart thumps furiously.

I stand abruptly. 'I need some fresh air. Let's walk outside.' I steady myself while my hands hover protectively over the growing abdomen in front of me. I ask him more questions as we walk, oblivious to the peering adolescent eyes through the classroom windows.

The breeze evaporates my cold sweat. Jon tells me that the most serious effects occur in foetuses under three months. I'm over that. I feel confused, torn between loyalties. If my child should suffer, how would I prevent the rage from subsuming me? In helping a friend, I jeopardise the health of my baby. Is this disease a scourge from God after all?

I live a nerve-wracking week waiting for the results of a blood test. My obstetrician had been quite positive and tells me over the telephone that I haven't got CMV but that I must avoid very close contact with Jon.

Yet, even as I tell Jon this, and he sighs with relief, I want to hug him. I don't want to increase his sense of alienation. But he begins to stand away from me whenever we're together and refuses to touch me or discuss coming to live with us.

He decides he'll go to Sydney as soon as the term ends. He needs AZT regularly and it's more readily available there. He believes he'll soon need blood transfusions and will get these if he goes in to the St Vincent's Hospital AIDS clinic. He needs to leave me so I can concentrate on the more essential issues in my life. I explode when he says this to me, but he smiles and whispers, 'It's meant to be.'

15

'KEVIN'S COMING TO GET ME at the end of term, two weeks from now. I told him about the way I'm living and he said why don't I just throw them out, cat litter and all. But he doesn't understand loneliness. If I should die in the middle of the night, who'll be there? I don't want to be alone because I don't want to die on my own. He asked about my other friends, gay friends. I tell some about what I've got and I don't hear from them again. My disease confronts them with things they don't want to think about. I can't rage at parties. I can't drink or engage in three-hour witty dinner conversation, so I'm not exactly popular anymore. Some care. But I need hospital treatment now. I have to face it.'

'Kevin'll be there for you in Sydney.'

'Yes.' Jon smiles. 'He keeps telling me he's going to harass me and nag me until the end.'

By December, Jon is hardly teaching. He has requested and been given a year of leave in 1988. His job will wait for him in 1989, if he should want to or be able to return.

It begins to dawn on me that soon he won't be around anymore. I won't see him daily, and I don't know when I'll see him again. I tell Jon I'm going to miss him. He says he knows he'll miss me, and will really hate missing the birth of the baby. But we'll see each other again, he assures me. 'I won't be able to stay away from you or Adelaide forever.'

My heart aches for him as I watch him walk slowly around the schoolyard, surrounded by students. He maintains a ready smile, but his witty retorts and hilarious questions are few. As the school year draws to a close, I watch him struggle to write student reports, stopping often to reflect and gaze out the window. The principal has told him he can leave any time. Someone else will write his reports. Jon adamantly refuses. 'I want to see this year out. I may never see these kids again. But I can't think clearly. I'll get them done somehow. If only my depression wasn't swallowing my mental ability. At least, I hope it's depression. I'm so scared of losing my mind.'

He sits alone in the staff-room, writing so slowly, his face mottled and gaunt. At times, I need to get up and walk out before he sees me lose control. At times he catches my frowns and whispers, 'Say something funny!'

Matteo arrives in Adelaide, bubbly and delighted after almost a year of travelling in Europe and the Americas. He has learned a new language, is considering beginning a Diploma in Business Studies, and wants to embark upon a new, 'serious' career. He arranges a get-together, specifically asking Jon to attend.

Jon decides he will go. 'I've got this morbid curiosity to see if I can pass a test. He hasn't seen me since the beginning of the year. I want to know what he'll say.'

'Why put yourself through this? You'll know what he'll say.'

'I want to see if he's still interested despite the way I've aged.'

Jon is accompanied to the Italian restaurant in Rundle Street by Sandra, a gentle, softly spoken college friend. Matteo has saved a seat for Jon next to him. As someone mentions they've arrived, he scans the door with a beaming face, but the smile becomes uncertain, and a slight frown lines his tanned forehead.

He shakes Jon's hand, searching his lowered eyes, and then helps him to the seat. A few pleasantries and then he says, 'You've lost so much weight. You look sick. Are you all right?'

I stare into my glass of mineral water, remembering the effort Jon has made to dress well. He's even been to a hairdresser to have his hair done.

Maria comments on Jon's hair, saying the shorter cut makes him look younger. 'I guess it doesn't accentuate my thinning hair,' Jon says. He looks over to me. 'Do I look younger, Maria?'

'Yes, you do, actually.' He does. He looks like a young, terribly ill man.

Under Matteo's questions, I see Jon's facade crumble and, in the next two hours, he says very little. He avoids talking to Matteo but listens without expression to his travel stories and plans.

As coffees are ordered, Jon stands to leave. 'You've hardly eaten!' Matteo says, rising with him.

'Not very hungry tonight.'

Matteo puts a hand on his shoulder. 'I'm sorry I went on about how skinny you look. I haven't seen you for so long. I'll ring you tomorrow.'

'I'm quite busy packing, moving to Sydney.'

'Really! To be with Kevin?'

'Not quite. I just want a year away from work and, in Sydney, I'll be able to catch up with old friends. What if we contact each other there?'

'Okay. Fine. I know where Kevin's living. I'll ring you.' Matteo takes his hand.

Jon farewells everyone and walks out.

After coffees, we go for a *passegiata* along the sidewalks of Rundle Street. Matteo takes my arm and we walk ahead of the others. He questions me about Jon, and I make my usual vague comments. He isn't satisfied but decides to pursue it no further, especially since I keep breaking into conversation about my pregnancy.

Towards the end of the evening, he tries again. 'Wasn't December the second Jon's birthday?'

'Yes.'

'What kind of outrageous gathering did he have?'

'None.'

'But he turned thirty, the beginning of a new decade.'

On Jon's thirtieth birthday, we sat and chatted, mulling over the issues and plans. Kevin would come to collect him on the tenth. Sydney was his only hope now. He was positive that with the much needed treatment he'd get better. 'I want to see some of my thirties even though my fortieth birthday will be celebrated in some other dimension.'

He looked at me and smiled, rubbing his bony fingers over my 'beer-gut', feeling for moving limbs. 'Look at you. And you're going to get fatter. What will I do without you around?'

I promised to write often and he made me promise to telephone as soon as the baby was born and to let him know all the 'gory details'. I made him promise to come over and see the baby in 1988. 'I'll bring my drips and transfusions and wheelchair and whatever else, but I'll definitely be here.'

He promised to return to live in Adelaide in 1989 if all went well. 'I've got strong hopes. I'll fight this to the end.'

'I wish it wasn't Sydney you were putting your hopes in.'

'Still got that funny phobia? I'll need to be there. Hey! You've got a new life in here.' He prodded my abdomen. 'It's going to be a busy 1988 for you, full to the brim. You wouldn't have much room for me, and that's the way it should be. From Sydney I'll be able to hear about your conquests and picture you studying away with a little woggy baby. I'll really treasure your constancy. It'll be my beacon.'

'Jon, forget the CMV. Let me hug you.'

'Well, actually, I've beaten the CMV.' We held each other close. Then, he drew me away, holding my shoulders at arms' length. 'Just in case some other little nasty's hovering about, and in case I never want to let go, let's just play safe.' His eyes twinkled.

Matteo is still arm-in-arm with me, strolling along Rundle Street. 'He had a good birthday,' I say.

16

DECEMBER TENTH ARRIVES, and Jon is not at work. I assume he's going to be late. I haven't seen him for two days because he's been ill, but I was sure he'd make an appearance today to say goodbye to everyone.

As the morning wears on, and he doesn't appear, I become more frantic. There is a barbecue scheduled for the staff in the afternoon, after the students have raced out of the school gates.

During morning recess, I ring him. 'What are you doing? Why aren't you at school? I want to say goodbye.'

'I don't want to say goodbye,' he says hoarsely.

'You can't just leave.' My voice chokes me.

'Kevin's coming to school with two letters, one for you and one for the staff. Please read it to them for me. I can't face the day there. I couldn't stand to be with you, knowing what we've been through. I'm scared I'll never see you or the school again.'

He pauses and I hear sounds of weeping. Then he continues, 'I'm going to live till I see you again, okay, in the middle of next year. After that, I'll live until I see you in February 1989. Back at the school together, okay? After that it'll get better and better, and we'll be looking back and laughing about 1988. Maria, I'm going to believe this.'

'Optimism of the will. I won't let you do it any other way.' My mouth trembles. 'I want to say so much.'

'You've said it all in many ways. Please understand.'

'I do. All right, I won't say goodbye. I'll see you here in the middle of next year and then I'll see you in February 1989, and we can begin back at this place together. You'd better not let me down. And keep writing!'

'You know I will. I'll still need to talk to you, so I'll do my talking on paper.' A pause. 'Please read my letter to the staff.'

'I'll try, Jon. But I don't know if I'll be strong enough.'

'You'll have to be strong about speaking on my behalf one day. You might as well practise.' He tries to laugh.

'I'll do it.'

I hear his heavy breathing before he speaks again. 'I'm going to hang up.'

'All right.'

And he does.

About half an hour later, Kevin arrives with the two letters. He doesn't want to see anyone so we're soon walking back to the red Mazda RX7. I run my fingers along the side of the car, hot and shimmering under the summer sun. I recall the days when the three of us zoomed around in it – loud music, loud laughter. I recall the drive home from Sydney.

'Take care of him, Kevin. He needs you. He still loves you.'

'I will. I do love him. I always have. But you understand, don't you?'

We hug. A few more words. By three that afternoon, Jon and Kevin will be somewhere on the road to Sydney, to proper treatment at St Vincent's.

The car zooms away.

At my own desk, with no one around, I read Jon's letter to me and then hide in the toilet until I've composed myself.

At the thought of the summer holiday stretching lazily ahead, the staff exuberantly enjoy the food and wine. I try to feel jovial, but the food sticks in my throat.

After several speeches from the principal and the staff members who are leaving, I stand up and, summoning all my strength, read Jon's simple letter. The teachers laugh at his usual mischievous humour: 'I guess I had to do something to get out of the four-day staff conference'; and reflect silently upon his genuine thanks for their friendship, good wishes for their futures, and his intention of 'inflicting' himself on everyone again in 1989.

A few days later, a Christmas card arrives from Kevin. It is a photograph of a tanned, muscular man with angels' wings and silky cloth wrapped alluringly around his waist. He holds a long, shiny gold clarinet. 'Hark the herald angel sings,' says the card. There is no message from Jon. He doesn't send a card.

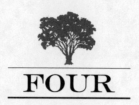

FOUR

Made weak by time and fate, but strong in will,
To strive, to seek, to find, and not to yield.

Alfred, Lord Tennyson

17

IT'S THE FIRST DAY of July 1988, and Jon is back in Adelaide. I drive along in my red Fiat, listening to its deep sounds, feeling excited and apprehensive. It has been a very different first half of the year for him, and for me.

Rob and I lugged our suitcases upstairs in our stiflingly hot house. We had just returned from a week's holiday in Melbourne, the company's reward for Rob's achievements. I lay on the bed for awhile, thinking about his career and my coming year away from work. The baby lunged around contentedly inside me.

Downstairs, Rob made us cool drinks and I opened my mail. There was a letter saying I'd been accepted into the Graduate Diploma of Arts in Women's Studies, and a letter from Jon.

'He sounds okay,' Rob said, when I read the letter to him.

I nodded, and smiled. Jon had been camping at Forster. 'Kevin took care of all my medical supplies and even managed to set my drip up without any complications,' he wrote. 'It only has to run into my veins for an hour and then I'm free for the rest of the day. He's very good – went straight in without any pain, bruising or second tries.'

He talked about buying a small unit somewhere near St Vincent's Hospital. It would give him the stability, the interest, the privacy, and a clean break from Kevin who had set up a new relationship with a man named Terry. 'In so many ways, Kevin and I were not suited, but I still love him.'

The moods in the letter continued to swing. He'd got my photos and commented how 'radical' I looked, huge, in bikinis on the beach and how depressing it was to get back to Sydney from Forster to face Kevin and Terry, his father's deteriorating health, lack of money, adjusting to a pension, living with four other people, the loss of career, what to do with the dog, and the fears and frustrations of his disease.

When I finished reading, Rob took the letter from me and read it again to himself. I looked at the neat, large handwriting, feeling the baby doing somersaults inside me.

18

I OFTEN PAUSED when I was reading Jon's letters to puzzle over the contradictions. Was he well? Was he sick? I had a feeling he was protecting me, struggling with what he should and shouldn't say.

The six-hourly AZT doses were giving him nausea and headaches and making him feel weak. The drug was hard on the body cells as well as on the viruses and could damage the liver and bone marrow, but he supposed it helped to prolong his life so he was prepared to give it a try.

He'd been to the Australia Day Bicentenary celebrations – music had always been his way of sounding his emotions – and the finale of the 1812 Overture, the stirring burst of cannon fire, the bells of St Mary's tolling, and the night skies lit up with fireworks had all matched his inner turmoil.

He talked about old college friends with whom he could reminisce, but said he missed his job and most especially Adelaide.

I visited the school, conscious of my protruding abdomen. It was exhilarating to be back among students, answering their questions and exchanging witticisms.

'Hey, you're back already.' Michael came up to me in the staff-room, a broad smile on his handsome face. We kissed each other and sat down. I realised I really missed him, and it wasn't only the daily parade of fashionable gear, the stylish walk, and silly jokes. 'I think a lot of us are missing you and Jon,' he said. 'Jon with his lunchtime crap-sessions, and you in your test-pattern clothes. Yeah, it's not the same.' Michael looked at me. 'You brightened things up around here.'

His voice was deep and throaty, the way it had been when Jon had told him the news.

'Hey, Maria,' Michael had called, beckoning me towards him. We were behind the science laboratories. No one else was around. His eyes had looked red, hurt, but he was defiant and angry. 'Jon's just told me he's got AIDS. You've known for a couple of months. Why didn't you tell me?'

'He didn't want me to tell anyone.'

'Didn't he think he could trust me, or something?' His hands had clasped together at the back of his neck. He lowered his head.

'What makes you angry? Not being told or Jon having AIDS?'

'It's so unfair,' he'd muttered. 'Why did this have to happen to him? Did he think I would broadcast the information?'

'Do you know,' Jon had told me 'one evening Kevin, Michael and I went for drinks in a gay pub. Michael had a few too many, and then, in this raucous voice, he yelled at me, 'Hey Jon, you poofter, come here!' I saw thunderbolts strike him from the eyes of every other poofter in the place.' Jon had burst into laughter. 'I've often told him he doesn't need to drink to express an emotion.' He'd snorted. 'God, I sound like my old college pastor. Michael's a sensitive man hiding behind a cool ocker.'

'Simone and I went to Sydney to see Jon and Kevin during the holidays,' Michael said, looking around him to see that no one was listening. 'Jon's quite jovial about his daily hospital journeys and being sick every day. Sim gets upset after she's been with him, but I keep telling her it's not going to be any use falling apart. He's all right.'

Jim walked up and gripped my shoulder as he sat down. He didn't know yet. Jon worried that he'd get distraught. He had reacted angrily and emotionally enough at the thought that Jon had cancer. 'So how's our man? Heard from him lately?'

I answered vaguely, using the set phrases for school visits.

19

IN MARCH, I TRIED to organise Jon's licence and sent him the forms. He sent them off with his ID and money so he now had his new South Australian driver's licence that was valid until 1993. 'They're thinking positively about me being around until then so maybe I should be too?' he wrote in his next letter. 'They don't know, do they?'

He now had a part-time job: two year eleven biology classes between recess and lunch each day so that he had time to get to the hospital and relax in the afternoon.

I felt relieved as I read how he was slowly regaining his old ground, looking outwards, involving himself in events and people around him. 'There are 1,100 boys crammed into a pocket handkerchief piece of land about one-tenth the area of my previous school. It's very inner city, richly ethnic, with Lebanese, Asian and aggressive Irish students. I'm sure there are at least three other gay teachers, but not one of us says anything. The woman whose desk is next to mine, and who I find myself talking to most of the time, is a twenty-eight-year-old Italian called Maria. She's been there for seven years and is an English/History teacher. I can't escape them.'

He bought himself a unit close to both the hospital and Kevin's place so that he would be able to take Sven for walks and drop in to see Kevin and Robbo when he needed company. He planned to re-paint and re-carpet, and regretted he couldn't carry out the renovations himself. He called his new home a 'punit' for it was so small, and his only concern was whether the stairs would prove an obstacle later.

He was looking forward to having his parents over in Sydney. It had been nearly eight months since he'd told them his news. Now he hoped to show them how well established he was. His sister, her husband and two children from Africa had been in Sydney for the past few weeks.

Now, all he needed was someone special: 'It's a basic part of human existence, isn't it? It's not so easy to find someone when your looks and vitality are on the slide, and you're in the grip of a terminal illness. Maybe I'll get a chance to chat up the person in the bed beside me when I'm in hospital.'

I missed him. I would feel anger gnaw at me as I thought about how things would've been without AIDS.

Jon's break with Kevin was harder than he had expected. 'It was when it came to sorting out the little things that I became depressed. I still keep finding things of his from time to time, like all our snow-gear tucked away in an old suitcase. I had to sort out his gloves, beanie, scarf, goggles, woollen socks, and long underpants. To cheer myself up, I went out and bought a piano, a brand new shiny little Beale. I've been playing and practising for a couple of hours every day, probably driving the other residents mad. I used up all my money buying it, but I decided I needed it now.'

The AZT was working – 'at one thousand dollars a bottle there should be miracles' – but there were some signs that it was beginning to attack the blood-producing cells in his bone marrow and he'd soon have to start having transfusions.

The letters continued, backwards and forwards, full of news. On Kevin's birthday, Jon enjoyed a night of feasting and dancing and had even had a little alcohol. He had been able to help Gary and Linda paint their place. There was only a hint of AZT-related difficulties, until June: 'I'm coming to Adelaide with Kevin next month to tie up my "loose ends".'

I felt alarm grow in me. He was shouting out to me between his controlled phrases. 'Today has been my first sickie all year, but I'm not any sicker than usual. I thought I had adapted to feeling tired and nauseated most of the time, with the odd headache and bouts of diarrhoea just to liven things up periodically. But, for some reason, I just couldn't get myself to work today.'

20

I GRIP THE STEERING WHEEL as I drive to pick him up. A whimper, like that of a kitten, comes from the backseat of my car. Three-month-old Stephanie is stirring in her sleep, snugly wrapped in the baby capsule. At the next red light, I turn to look at her. She's asleep again, her little pink hands, her tiny nails visible. The car smells of her baby freshness. Jon will be seeing her for the first time.

On March the twenty-ninth, Stephanie decided it was time to be born. In giving birth to her, I faced pain so agonising that I was on the verge of panic, had to struggle to control it. Rob held me, coaxed me through the pounding waves.

When they subsided and I floated to the surface, I wondered at the pain others must live with, must die in. At least I knew I wouldn't die, and that at the end of the battering there would be a new life.

We were like children, Rob and I, marvelling at this two handfuls of humanity. She wriggled gently, eyes staring unseeing into our eyes. Our minds and hearts journeyed into her future, inextricably linked to ours. There was a measured portion of earthly time ahead of her, but no one knew how much. Gazing at the smooth round face, the tiny fingers, the little perfectly formed body wrapped securely in a white blanket, I wept to think that one day this life we'd given would be extinguished, and it made me think of Jon and his parents. I resolved to make the most of my relationship with Stephanie, to do my best not to let differences of attitude get in the way.

Soon after Stephanie was born, Rob had phoned Jon. I wanted to speak to him too, but I was exhausted and afraid I'd cry.

'What did he say?' I asked as soon as Rob returned, his face beaming. He smoothed wisps of my hair away from my face as he spoke. 'He sends you his hugs and kisses and says welcome to motherhood. He can't wait to hold the little Maria when he comes to Adelaide.' Rob reached over and cupped his huge paw gently around Stephanie's head. 'He got a bit choked up at the end. He was about to say something, but then said he had to hang up.'

I spent a sunny afternoon out on my balcony, the baby sleeping next to me in her bassinette, writing the 'gory details' to Jon.

'I went to bed before midnight on Monday with a slight backache, which I put down to my typically hectic day. But I woke about midnight with pains in my abdomen. I began to time them and counted three about ten minutes apart, so I woke Rob, who was up like a flash, locking the windows, getting dressed, getting my bags, while I sat up in bed watching him, wondering, and timing my contractions.

'We listened to some of our favourite music, kept timing contractions, and just talked for about two hours.

'Finally, my waters broke and I rang the hospital, both sets of parents, Maria and Mike, and other friends who wanted to know as soon as I went in.

'It was funny driving to the hospital in the dead of night. I felt excited and nervous, whispering a farewell to our home and wondering what would've happened by the next time I saw it.

'Between two and six, my contractions ranged from ten minutes to five minutes. My parents had come in to the hospital and spent a few hours with us before going to the waiting-room. It felt strange and yet beautiful having my Mum and Dad there, watching my pain and listening to my ramblings. And when I nodded off, I would wake to their teary smiling faces.

'Rob was great. I tried to put all my ante-natal classes into practice – breathing, relaxation, massage, mind-power – and we walked around a lot to speed up the opening of the cervix. My mother couldn't believe it. She'd been confined to her bed during her deliveries.

'At six, my friend Maria came in. She said there was no way she could go to work without spending time with me. She made me laugh so much because she couldn't believe that one moment I was in excruciating pain that she said she could feel, and next, while my white gown got more and more stained, I'd be carrying on some reflective conversation about feminism and mothering.

'At eight, Rob's brother's girlfriend came in with her Mum. Maria looked like she could feel my pain too.

'By ten, the pains were about three minutes apart and getting stronger so we went back to the labour room. I kissed my parents and told them it wouldn't be long.

'I began to use the gas mask, squeezing Rob's hand every time a contraction started, as if by doing that I could stop myself from losing control and panicking when I was lost in this terrifying sea of gas and pain.

'By noon, the baby was pushing at my cervix and I felt as if my spine was breaking, my bowels splitting, and yet I didn't panic or swear or scream. I "rode" the pain and was given a dose of pethidine.

'Not long after, the midwife announced it was time to get the obstetrician, and thank goodness, he poked his head around the door just then because Stephanie was coming through fast.

'I was watching in the mirror and I remember the midwife holding the head in as the sheets were arranged beneath me. My whole body seemed to have gone into its own motion of pushing – and by 12.31 pm Stephanie was out. I can't describe how we felt! We were left alone with her for some time until a nurse came in looking worried. She said our families wanted to come in, but we didn't have to let them in if we didn't want the confusion. We giggled. She obviously didn't understand how thrilling it would be to have our families there to see Stephanie before she got all cleaned up. So Rob's parents, my parents, and my aunt and uncle came pouring in. The men were particularly inter-ested in Stephanie, who continued to suckle away throughout the inspection and noise. In their time, they'd never seen a new-born, yukky and mottled. But I don't know how much my father could see behind the film of tears in his eyes.

'The mothers kept saying they couldn't believe I was already so energetic, chatting and smiling away. I tried to explain that I'd been in control and understood every step. It hadn't been like their experiences where language barriers, fear because they didn't understand what was happening to them, and arrogant male doctors who treated them like cows, had made it a nightmare.

'On the following Sunday night, Stephanie had her first Easter party with our families. We had told everyone we'd be out on Monday, hoping to surprise the clan by our sudden arrival at Tony and Eva's place.

'It looks like Rob is going to make a great parent. He knows how to do everything – except breastfeed. If he had his way, he'd probably arrange for that to happen too, and if there were a way, he'd have the next one. I said that'd be all right by me.

'And that's the whole story. I wish you had been here.'

Stephanie is still sleeping as I leave her in the car, parked in the driveway outside the trendy unit where Jon's friend lives.

Steve welcomes me in. 'Jon's just getting his gear organised. Excuse the chaos in here, but friends stayed over until the small hours.' I step into the very tidy lounge, and stir him about needing to wade through the filth. I laugh loudly, hoping Jon can hear my voice.

'I'd better check on Steph,' I say.

Steve's eyes widen and he whispers, 'Does Jon know she's with you?'

I shrug and hurry out. I'm beginning to feel nervous.

Stephanie is still fast asleep so I hurry back in just as Jon is emerging from the hallway.

For a moment, I am taken aback. He looks paler, thinner, hesitant and vulnerable. He stops moving when he sees me, and leans back slightly against the hallway wall, fists plunged deeply into his jacket pockets, shoulders hunched. His blue eyes seem larger, rounder. He looks at me, waiting.

My mind rewinds and I see the image of my old friend superimposed. I move forward to embrace him, his arms rising slowly to encircle me. Beneath my palms, I feel the rib-cage, his spine, his bony shoulder blades.

'It's so good to see you.' I move back to look at him but hold his hands.

Jon nods, slowly. His eyes, which smile nervously at me, seem glazed. 'Yes. It hasn't been long. It seems . . . quite a time.' His voice is hoarse. 'I guess, well, I've changed, haven't I?' He searches my eyes.

I place my hands on my hips, bend my head to one side, and pretend to scrutinise him through squinting eyes. 'Have you? For better or worse? Let me know what I'm in for. I've had a long holiday from your rabble-rousing. I might've lost my touch.'

Jon laughs. It is so good. 'For worse, I think. I'm becoming quite unbearable.' His shoulders have relaxed.

Steve clears his throat. 'I hate to break this up, but what about – ' and he points outside, 'that package in the car.'

I cup my hands over my mouth and we break into laughter. 'I'd forgotten.'

Jon's smile widens into a grin and his eyes light up. 'The baby! You've got the baby.' He moves past us, out through the front door, and by the time we've stepped outside, he's pressed against the back sidewindow of the car, looking in at Stephanie. 'So peaceful,' he whispers.

'Believe me, she has her loud, unpeaceful moments.'

'Well, she's your daughter, what do you expect?'

'Oh, here we go again.' I punch his arm.

We drive home, talking constantly. Our voices are hushed, conscious of the baby behind us, and the quiet car, with the muffled sounds of outside traffic, is warm and cosy.

At home, Jon insists on carrying his bags in. But in the hallway, he puts them down abruptly, and breathes heavily. I put Stephanie's capsule on the lounge. As he moves towards her, I duck back into the hall, pick up his bags, and race upstairs with them.

When I come back, Jon is still standing near the capsule, looking down at the baby, hands in pockets. He turns to me. 'Have you got a heater? I get cold easily. I'm sorry, I don't mean to be a nuisance.'

I get a heater and set it up near his feet. He sits directly in front of it, thin wiry hands outstretched while I warm some milk for him. He sips it slowly and quizzes me about what he calls my 'adventures in academia'.

Now and again, he glances at Stephanie. He yawns,

stretching the pallid skin over his cheekbones. 'I need an afternoon nap, but I want to see Stephanie awake first.'

'She's due to wake for lunch.' But even as I speak, Stephanie wakes up and starts whimpering. Jon walks over to the capsule, his hands reaching out to her and then retreating to his pockets.

I pick her up and hold her out to him as he talks about her dark eyes and dark hair. He doesn't touch her.

'Just hold her for me while I fix her lunch,' I say quickly and deposit the baby in his arms which have come up instantly to receive her, a nervous smile on his face. I turn around and walk out into the kitchen. Don't cry, Stephanie, please don't cry. I take my time to mash some banana and blend it with baby cereal. I listen to the silence wafting out from the lounge-room. And then I hear soft endearments.

When I walk back in, he's sitting near the heater, cradling her in his arms, his forefinger clenched in her fist. 'She's gorgeous. Look how she holds my finger.'

'She likes her Uncle Jon.' A dull ache begins inside me.

'What an interesting human being you're going to be.'

Stephanie interrupts him with a cry of hunger, and turns her head into his breast.

Jon laughs in delight and hands her to me.

I unbutton my shirt and begin to breastfeed. Jon sits back into the lounge next to me, watching and smiling. 'So here you are, actually a mother.'

'I may be a mother now but I'm still Maria. It's an important part of my life, not my whole life.'

Jon giggles. 'And I once thought you weren't a feminist.'

Eventually, Stephanie nods off again and Jon rises. 'I must sleep. I want to be fresh and alert when I meet everyone here tonight. I'm such a baby too, you see. I need my naps.' He takes the heater with him to the spare bedroom.

Dinner is a hot minestrone soup, with warm bread and good conversation, as Rob and Jon catch up with each other.

'We both seem to be losing our blonde locks,' Jon says.

'I'm losing my hair and putting on weight,' Rob replies.

'Give me some,' Jon says and pinches Rob's waist.

'Wish I could!' There is much talk of medications and drips and viruses.

Jon eats sparingly, and then sits in the lounge-room waiting for his friends. He fidgets nervously. A fire is roaring in the fireplace and it lights his troubled face with a rosy glow.

When we hear a knock on the door, Jon says, 'Maria, please tell Jim tonight. I don't think I can tell him myself.'

I ask Jim to help me get the next round of drinks in the kitchen. 'Jon doesn't look well at all,' he says quietly.

'He wants me to tell you something. But you mustn't tell anyone, except Katrina. Michael and Simone know. He wants you to carry on as normal with him.'

Jim looks at me intently. 'He's got AIDS,' I say.

Jim frowns, shuts his eyes tight, the circles underneath them reddening. He thumps a fist on the bench. 'I think I've always known.' His voice falters. 'When he told me he had lymphoma, I knew there was more. But it was all right that he didn't want to say.' He wipes his eyes with the palms of his hands. 'But you know the exact moment it was confirmed for me? Tonight, when Perry arrived. Perry bent to kiss Jon's hand, since he's taken over Jon's position. Before Jon would let him, he looked carefully at the back of his hand to see if there were any cuts.' I put an arm around his shoulders.

He gives his eyes a final wipe. 'He's more of a man to me than any of those dickheads that go around poofter-bashing.'

We return to Jon's gathering, too many cool drinks juggled precariously in our hands.

Just past midnight, Jon sinks deeper into his chair and says very little. He struggles to smile cheerily, attempts the occasional witty comment, but prefers to observe from a misty distance.

Friends begin to leave. It's time to say goodbye again. Jon handles it well, promising to be back early in February 1989. Simone buries her tearful face in his shoulder. Michael clasps his hand in both of his but maintains his jovial control. Jim reaches over and enfolds Jon's thin body in his solid one. 'Take bloody good care of yourself, mate. Remember, you're the one whose canoe never seemed to capsize while the rest of us were the shit-scared drowning rats.'

Rob stokes the fire, and I begin to clear away the glasses. Jon stretches out on the lounge, knees pulled up towards him, his hands clasped between them, eyes shut, breathing deeply. Rob puts a blanket over him.

He wakes in a few minutes but lies silently on his side. I sit on the edge of the lounge in front of him, massaging his shoulder. 'Did I put on a good performance?' he asks, and smiles wryly.

'You did fine. You made it very easy for all of us. You stirred us and had us all laughing like you used to.'

'Yes, it was good. I'm glad I've seen them again.'

'You'll see them again next year,' Rob says.

Jon smiles, sits up slowly, swinging his feet to the floor. 'And Jim?'

'It's okay. He knew all along. He thinks you're a very courageous man.'

Jon stands and smiles again. 'I must go to bed. Thank you for the gathering. I'm tired and cold, despite that glorious fire.'

'There're more blankets in the cupboard, and towels. Call me if –'

Jon hugs me. 'There's a toilet next door, which will be extremely handy. I'll be right.'

Rob and I watch him climb the stairs, gripping the banister as he hoists himself forward.

At about eleven next morning, a windy, drizzly Sunday, we hear Jon shower and Rob sets off. We had decided it would be good if Jon and I could have some time together alone.

As Jon makes his way downstairs, I prepare his freshly squeezed orange juice. 'My morning ritual, although usually accompanied by medication,' he says as he takes the glass from me, and drinks it quickly.

I prepare some lunch for Stephanie and hear him play and talk with her. 'So what's it like having this woman for a mother? Is it bearable? I'm sure you'll teach her a thing or two. I do sympathise. She can be quite tyrannical – bewitching.'

I walk in to the lounge-room. He holds a finger to his lips, and whispers to Stephanie cuddled into his lap. 'Ssh, here she comes. What were you saying about bowel problems? You get constipated. Well, my dear, having diarrhoea every day is really no fun at all.'

As I feed her, Jon crouches near the open fire. 'Can we go for a drive?'

'It's disgusting weather outside. What if you catch something?'

'We'll be in the car, nice and warm. Red sports cars seem to be conducive for deep and meaningfuls, don't they?'

I nod, remembering our drive home from Sydney.

'I also need some stuff for my mouth. The fungal sores are coming up again.'

'Did you sleep well?'

'I blacked out as soon as I got into bed, mercifully. But the sheets were all saturated. I've left them on the bed. They'll be dry by now.'

I pack Stephanie into the baby capsule. She's just dozing off again. 'Well, we've got three hours before she wakes. Let's go touring.'

The wind rips at us as we step outside. Jon cowers into his jacket. It's a two-door car and he has to wait while I fix the contraption for Stephanie. I try to hurry. But he's laughing as he eventually sits in the car. 'It's hilarious! A baby capsule in a red hot sports car. A mother with Rastafarian long locks and black leggings driving an AIDS-riddled queen through the mellow streets of Adelaide.' He sucks in air.

I wait in the car outside the chemist. Jon hurries out, one hand behind his back, grinning sheepishly. I reach across and open his door. Quickly, he sits in the car, and holds out a clenched fist. 'For you,' he says shyly.

I pick it up out of his palm. It's a blue elephant, its trunk extended upwards, and perched on the end is a tiny white mouse. The inscription on the base reads, 'Friends Are Forever'.

Jon touches the figurine. 'It's us. I found it on a dusty shelf all by itself.'

'Oh, so who is the fat elephant?'

He pretends to examine my abdomen. But his voice is soft and serious. 'Well, I often feel like a white mouse.'

'Elephants are scared of mice.'

'You're not your average elephant.'

He squeezes some ointment out of the tube and with a forefinger rubs it on the inside of his mouth. He wheezes and puffs out air. 'It bloody stings!'

I look at the tube. It's the ointment recommended for teething babies.

Elephant and mouse on the dashboard and baby sleeping in the back, we visit Jon's old homes. The drizzling rain acts like a screen through which we must peer, as the landscapes of the past solemnly proclaim their link to us.

The memories are bittersweet. The establishing and nurturing of a relationship in one; the days of carefree neighbours blending into each other's lives and cultures in another; the dream home and entrepreneurial nightmares; the Unley villa where the chink in the relationship widens; the Sturt Street unit where AIDS finally drove him away to Sydney.

'This was it,' Jon says. 'The end of that saga.' He turns to me. 'Let's go to the beach.'

We park the car overlooking the grey expanse of water. The sky weeps, sprinkling the restless waves with tears. The roar of the ocean and the vibrations of the wind threaten the warm stillness in the car.

We sit, eating hot chips, looking out.

'I love the beach in winter,' Jon says.

'I don't like it. It depresses me.'

Jon smiles. 'I'm drawn to this. I sit along the cliffs in Sydney and watch the dark clouds hurrying on to war. I feel at home in all that fury.'

'Why?'

'Because I know that somewhere out there, in those infinite cycles of life and time, there is meaning in it all. It's bloody awful getting there, but once I've shed this troublesome flesh, I'll be free, at peace with myself, and powerful. Part of God's universe.'

'No longer afraid of death?'

'I'm afraid of the getting there, not being there. Albert Camus once wrote that we all have different ways of living. And we all have different ways of dying. So what? In the end, there'll be balance. My life hasn't been any more absurd than anyone else's. The various illusions we all construct ourselves within will be stripped away.'

We drive home silently. It's difficult to see the road as it blends with grey sky. I wonder how Jon sees the road.

Over the next two days, Jon, who is getting progressively weaker, catches up with other friends. He comes over with Kevin who shows us a new photo album: the American holiday, work, new friends, parties. And Terry. 'He's literally tall, dark and handsome,' I say. Jon snorts and nods.

I'm glad Kevin is feeling so self-assured. As he tells stories, Jon laughs scornfully. 'What a wide-eyed baby! I've been there, done that.'

'But I haven't,' I say. 'So keep talking!'

Lizzie holds a party for her brother the next evening so that Kevin is surrounded by his friends and family. Jon sits back in an old armchair, pointing out characters to Rob and me.

'See that couple?'

'Yes. Both stunning!' I follow his gaze.

'That one's HIV positive and that's his partner who loves him.'

'He looks so well.'

'He's determined to defeat it. He's emotionally secure, quit work, and they're off on a world tour next month.'

'You've travelled too, don't forget.'

'A comforting thought when I feel I can't tap into the life going on around me. I remind myself I was once in the centre of it all.'

'You were, and are, very significant in other's lives.'

'I'm more the dying man in the corner. Displaced.'

By midnight, Jon sits feebly, hands in pockets. His eyes follow Kevin.

He shivers despite the suffocating warmth in the room. 'Listen, I'm getting so cold, and I've been getting sick again – diarrhoea, fungal sores. I need to get back on AZT. So, I'm leaving tomorrow. Kevin's driving me. I need to get back to the hospital. I was too proud to lug my medicine cabinet with me to Adelaide.' He chuckles. 'I've got my niche and it might be best to stay there. You all have your lives in Adelaide, and for that I'm glad. But I'm not really part of it, which is how it should be now.' He laughs dryly. 'I feel like the withered old uncle here tonight.'

Soon, he decides to leave, and Rob and I drive him to his friend's unit where he's staying.

I step outside with him. 'When do I see you again?'

'If I'm well, I'll be back in February. But you may have to come and see me.'

'I will.'

Jon takes my hand in his. 'It would be wonderful to take you to Sydney with me. But you have an important life here.

'Keep writing to me.'

We cling to each other for a moment.

As the car begins to move forward, I can't help shouting, 'Take care of yourself!'

Jon smiles, a hand raised to say goodbye, the other holding his jacket closed in front of him.

21

EARLY IN AUGUST, Jon writes. He's had pneumocystis, and the Bactrim he's been on for ten days has given him fever, rashes, and maddening itching. He'd been on an intravenous drip of pentamidine for five days which made him nauseated and irritable. 'I used to wake up at three in the morning feeling angry and restless,' he writes.

He's beginning to develop serious side-effects as his liver and kidneys are subjected to heavy drugs and his system is being given a rest from AZT for a few weeks.

'One good thing about the Bactrim is that it cleared up my intestinal problems. I've been passing normal stools and farting with confidence for almost three weeks, one of life's simple joys.'

But he's going blind in his right eye owing to CMV retinitis. The doctors hope to be able to halt the disease by giving him DHPG injections into the affected eye. But because of scarring, he has permanent loss of vision. 'It's a bit frightening and sometimes I get so angry. I was a normal, capable healthy thirty-year-old man before AIDS reduced me to a fearful hypochondriac. I wonder what further insults are in store for me.'

He decides to sell his car, he reports that Matteo is 'going through boyfriends like toilet paper' and thoroughly enjoying his new job as 'an empty-headed, glamour-conscious fashion buyer', and speaks about his own work, saying that he's enjoying the challenge, the social contact, the pay cheque.

Matteo rings me. 'I've got business in Adelaide, and a family wedding. Let's get together. I want to talk.'

When he arrives at my place, he seems subdued, the flamboyance replaced by a brooding demeanour. I ask about his job, and he speaks rapidly and offhandedly. 'I couldn't face going back to Mount Gambier after my taste of the cosmopolitan life. I was going to take up more studies but I met the right people and got this great job.' He looks down at his hands, and then at me again. 'I know about Jon. You're a real friend, but I wish you'd told me.'

Matteo sits back. 'We began visiting each other's houses. One night we went out to the Albury for a drink. As we reached the corner of Surry and Victoria Streets where Jon turns off to go home, he said to me, "Matteo, I've got something to tell you. Come around tomorrow and we'll have a talk." I got all excited thinking he'd say, "Matteo, I want you. I've always wanted you!" I also thought to myself, he's a bit skinny but it's nothing my Italian cooking can't fix!'

Matteo looks at me wryly. 'That following night, Jon said, "This is something you've probably suspected for a while," and I'm thinking, Oh Jon, how sweet, but honestly I never guessed before now that you still wanted me. Jon continued, "You've been coming over quite a bit and we're getting on so well I can tell you're not some here-today, gone-tomorrow acquaintance. I feel I can trust you." I'm thinking, Wow! He's already proposing to me! But this is all so sudden! And then he just said, "Matteo, I've got AIDS." I felt like someone had slapped me for no reason. And I said, "Jon, you can't possibly have AIDS". You've had a boyfriend for hundreds of years and you don't do the sort of things that give you AIDS.' But he explained, and I realised this was no joke. So I said I'd help him in any way.'

Matteo's eyes fill with tears. 'I'd always hoped that one day Jon would need me, that I'd be cooking and cleaning for him. Well, my wish has come true. Sort of. I went to see him in hospital when he got back from Adelaide. He was hooked up to all sorts of contraptions.' He smiles. 'This AIDS thing has got me thinking, and being with Jon and planning to get a unit together and yet knowing he's not able to make long-term plans. Yeah, I've been thinking. I'm playing it safe, growing up, finally, you're probably thinking.' He leans over and squeezes my hand. 'I'd love to adopt a child. I don't want one-night stands and hangovers for the rest of my life. I've enjoyed myself in the past but what about when I'm old, when I lose my looks and the ability to catch any lover I want?

'Look, if I'm lucky enough to escape this AIDS bizzo, I want to redefine my life. I want a successful career. But I want someone to share a home with. I want real friends to talk to and love. I want a reliable partner who doesn't find another hunk to keep his bed warm while I'm away. But it's so hard. I've been in love so many times and really thought it'd last and then it fizzled out. I want stability and communication but I don't want to give up excitement. I'm scared of boredom and routine.'

We talk on. As he stands to leave, we hug each other tight. I feel an even greater warmth in our friendship.

'Kiss Jon for me,' I say. 'Take care of him.'

'Oh yes, I do that. He's trusting me with things, and I cook him a few wholesome pasta meals, but he's always making comments about how flighty I am and about my so-called boyfriends. I'd change tomorrow for the right person.'

Matteo leans out of the car window. 'There's one thing I keep thinking. When I first met Jon, I would've given anything for us to form a long-term relationship. If I'd succeeded I might have the virus now. I feel angry and sad. We could've started something. I could've made a real commitment to Jon. I love his mind, his character, and the way he likes the Italian in me. But that dream's dead.'

'Will you tell him how you feel?'

'I've thought about it, but it would just add to his pain.'

It is soon November. Matteo visits now and again, or rings, and tells me Jon is okay; and Jon writes and tells me he is surviving, 'despite one thing and another'. I think of him daily.

Michael and Simone had been to see him in the third-term break. His health has taken a sudden downturn, Michael reports. He is totally blind in his right eye, and losing weight and the muscular control in his arms and legs. 'But we took him out and made him laugh and had a great time. He's still a stirrer.'

'He hasn't been giving me many details in his letters.'

'Write to him and tell him we've spoken to you. He doesn't like dwelling on what's happening to him.'

For days, I think about writing a letter. Creating it in my mind. 'He's really interested in what you're doing, and your plans. He talked about you quite a bit,' Michael says.

I finally put pen to paper: 'My Mum has finished work. Well, not quite. I knew she'd never stop working completely. She'll be doing four hours on Saturday and Sunday mornings for pocket money and independence. She'll look after Stephanie next year.

'When I think of all the things my parents have been through, I get really emotional because my brother and I are reaping the benefits. We lead such comfortable, cushy lives. But they laugh and say they're extremely happy and feel really blessed because they've achieved what they set out to do, and now can take it easy and lavish their love on their grandchildren.

'You know, despite their irregular hours, they never neglected us. Emotionally, they were always there for us, even if physically they were not always accessible. But then there were my auntie and uncle and grandmother ready to step in.'

I stop writing, read back over what I have written. The words seem so superficial; the hopes and sentiments trivial compared to the words I want to write. I resume writing and the last paragraph tumbles out awkwardly.

'I know I still miss you. I find myself reminiscing about the fun we had together, the talks, the ideas, and then I think of the pain and disappointments I shared with you and wanted to take away from you. But I remember a lot of laughs, how much I have learned from you, and I know you are a great person.'

A week later, his letter arrives, proclaiming there's definitely something psychic between us: he's been thinking about me a great deal lately.

He talks about missing the school in Adelaide, and wanting me to keep him informed about the lives and doings of his friends there. 'At work, they still don't have any idea that there is anything wrong because they've only ever known me as skinny and unhealthy. They think I'm quiet and shy since I usually sit on my own at my desk in the corner of our massive staff-room. Hard to believe I don't gasbag, isn't it?'

He had just returned from a weekend at Avondale College. 'It was graduation weekend and some of the religious stuff was a bit nauseating, but walking around the campus and in the surrounding bush parklands brought back great memories. I got quite a kick out of seeing the massive trees at our old house which I had planted as a kid.

'I think my next birthday is worth celebrating considering what I've been through in the last twelve months. We're holding a banquet at Matteo's place.'

He looked forward to having his sister from Africa to stay with him for a week and then going away to spend Christmas with his parents. 'It'll be good to see them again.'

On the first day of December, Jon is thirty-one and I send him a birthday card. It depicts a sunny blue sky, a sunny blue ocean, and warm yellow sand. Two masculine feet can be seen just peeping from the edge of a bright umbrella. Inside, the printed message asks the reader to bask in the warmth and peace of a summer's day at the seaside.

I am plagued by unsettling memories of his predictions from the reading of his own palm. 'I won't live to see much of my thirties.'

A card arrives from Sydney. Kevin has written on one page, Jon on the other. I read Kevin's first.

'How things change. How's that beautiful Aries child of yours?'

I think of Kevin, an Aries, caught between his future and his past with Jon still such an important part of his life.

Jon's note sounds deceptively carefree. 'I don't know why I let that Kevin creature desecrate my card to you. I'm stuck in hospital so I thought I'd erase the boredom by getting my cards and letters done. I've become rather weak lately and they're dripping a whole new batch of blood into me. I have plenty of visitors and you'd love all the chocolates.'

Matteo returns to Adelaide to have an early Christmas weekend with his family. His department store has booked him into the Hilton. He rings to invite us to visit him in his suite. We laugh and joke as he takes us for a tour through the hotel. Back in his room, I ask about Jon.

Matteo shakes his head, smiling sadly.

'What's happening?'

Rob sits forward. 'We know he's been getting new blood. Has it helped?'

'He can't hold down much food and he always gets diarrhoea if he does get it down. His whole digestive system seems to be malfunctioning as well as his liver and kidneys, and he's losing the use of his arms.'

I look down at my hands. Matteo reaches out for me and grasps one of my wrists. 'He's trying so hard. I try to cook for him, spend time with him, and he puts up such a front. He's so strong! I really admire him. I love him. He still says some pretty tacky stuff to me about my life, but I refuse to get offended. I can imagine what he's going through.'

'Perhaps Jon cares for you more than he'd like to right now,' Rob says.

Matteo accepts that with a nod. He tells us about Jon's birthday party, the fun and laughter, the interesting mix of people. 'Jon's Adventist crowd and conservative gay crowd were terribly proper and restrained. My lot were loud and outrageous, screaming and dancing. Jon's friends couldn't understand the fuss about our dancing, or why I was wearing cycling shorts. But after a while, everyone got to know each other.'

He shows us a photograph. I stare at Jon's gaunt, feeble frame, his shoulders hunched, hands deep in jacket pockets, a fixed smile on his face. His hair is thinner, his eyes deeply shadowed. Matteo towers over him. Strong, healthy, an arm firmly arm around Jon's shoulders. Matteo is leaning towards him, Jon is leaning slightly away. Behind them, glass slide-doors and the lights of Sydney.

'Can I have this?'

'Yes,' says Matteo softly. He pulls me towards him, arm around my shoulders.

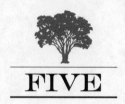

FIVE

Perhaps we've stopped a fleeting moment here
While on our way to quite another sphere.
Perhaps we must profoundly be debased
Before in honor elsewhere we'll be raised.
Perhaps our death which heightens all our fear
Will, with annihilation, turn to cheer.
Perhaps our lives are only obstacles
En route to where there are no earthly shackles.

Hjalmar Gullberg

22

I SIT BACK, anticipating the dread I always feel when planes take off, but this time I don't feel afraid at all. The fear has been supplanted by anxiety about what awaits me. I grin grimly. I could actually enjoy this flight. I look out and watch the sky darkening as we head into the warm Friday evening.

Michael had been to Sydney. 'Jon's pretty sick,' Michael told me at the first staff conference of 1989. 'He discharged himself from hospital in December because he said he was feeling okay, went off to Tasmania, and came back two weeks later thinner and sicker than ever. He got held at the airport on his way back because they thought he was some sort of drug addict. Interrogated for hours. Kevin said he could hardly walk when he was finally allowed to leave. Simone and I tried to take him out a bit. She cried all the time we were there. He thinks he'll get better again now that he's home.'

I felt a surge of panic and tried not to let it show as other friends began their routine questioning on Jon's situation. 'He's not well,' I found myself saying over and over again. I had forgotten the grind of the daily deception.

The woman sitting next to me in the plane is wearing a tailored black suit, her blonde hair neatly tied back with a black bow. I look down at my leggings, and my lime-green shirt, which is really Rob's. My hair creates its own dishevelled patterns around me.

I look at her ear-rings, delicate little diamond drops. I reach up to my multi-coloured, hand-painted wooden ones. She catches my gaze, smiles placidly at me, reaches down into her briefcase and takes out a book. Medicine? Business? I'm curious. It's a book on mysticism, spiritualism, and the experiences of people who have 'crossed to the other side'.

I look out the window.

I rang Jon in the last few days of January, just after the first term had got underway. I knew what I wanted to say but not how to say it. It was a strange, distant conversation that took place.

'Michael told me you're not very well. How are you?'

His answers were short, and his voice sounded hollow, as if someone had sucked the spirit out of him.

'What do the doctors say?'

'Nothing, really.'

'What about medication?'

'I have to keep taking it.'

There was a pause. My voice was beginning to waver. 'I'm thinking of coming over in late February. I'll ask for the time off next week so the boss has plenty of warning.'

'If you can. But I'm doing all right, really.'

'But Michael said –'

'He hadn't seen me for a while.'

Another pause.

'How are you?' he asked.

'Okay.'

'What's your latest achievement?'

'It's working out like you said it would. But I keep two feet on the ground.' I bit my lower lip and kept the mouth-piece at a distance.

'How's Rob?'

'Great.'

'And your beautiful daughter?'

'Great. Full of life – too much sometimes.' I tried to laugh.

He did not laugh. 'She must be really growing up now.'

'Yes, she's changing. We might bring her with us when we come over to see you.'

'That would be nice.'

That frustrating politeness.

'Jon? Can I do anything for you?'

'Not really. I'll keep trying to pick up.'

'You're a survivor.'

'Yes.'

'Take care of yourself.'

He was breathing heavily. 'I have to go. Kevin's here. He's cooked some food for me.'

'Smell good?'

'I can't smell much anymore. That's better, I guess. I can't complain about the sludge I'm fed.'

'I bet Kevin takes good care of you.'

'Yes. He's always about. Can't get rid of him. And Robbo. Cleaning up my messes.'

He coughed slightly and said again, 'I must go. It's been good talking to you. I don't know when I'll get a chance to write. My arm's not that strong anymore.'

'What have you done about work?'

'Oh, I resigned. Why work?'

I knew how much teaching meant to him.

'I must go and have something to eat.'

'I don't want to hang up.' My throat narrowed. I swallowed and let the words rush out. 'Jon, I don't know what to say. I mean, I miss you. So much. I love you heaps!'

'It's all right. I know. I love you heaps. I'm journeying, remember?'

I thought about our conversation at the beach on the cold day in July when he came to Adelaide.

'Goodbye.'

'I'll see you at the end of next month.'

'If you can. Bye.'

Neither of us hung up. Jon spoke again. 'I'm going to hang up.'

'Okay,' and as the receiver was put down hastily, I sat in my hallway, recalling the last time he had told me he'd hang up.

Rob's hands caressed my shoulders, gently moving me away from the telephone.

Kevin telephoned me the next evening. 'I think you should know,' he began in a slow, measured voice, 'Jon's very sick. I could hear him last night talking to you. He wasn't telling you everything.'

'What is it? What's he hiding?'

'How sick he really is. He has a walking stick now. He can't go up and down stairs to his unit anymore. Robbo has to carry him. He's beginning to lose his hearing.'

'Oh, Kevin. Why won't he tell me?'

'He hurts talking to you. He got off the phone and sat on the floor crying. 'She's got her own life' he kept saying. 'But I wish she was here.' And he couldn't eat. He just sat in his chair staring at the wall.'

'I'll come over.'

'That'd be fantastic. The doctors don't think he's got long. Another month or two.' Kevin's voice faded away.

'Oh no.' I buried my eyes in my hand.

'Poor Jonno. He's fighting it, but it's fighting him too. He's lost his bladder control, and sometimes his bowel control, and he gets so humiliated, angry and scared.'

'What about you? How are you coping?'

'All right. But it takes its toll.' His voice faded away. We wept on either end of the line. 'I think we'll all be looking forward to seeing you.

23

THE FLIGHT STEWARD brings us our trays. The woman next to me eats daintily. I eat nervously. I think about why I'm going to Sydney and wonder whether I will be of much use to Jon. Perhaps sharing some wonderful memories. Perhaps just saying thank you to him in some way.

I had bought Jon a Valentine Card the day after I rang him. I was drawn to a bright red one with a white crescent moon. From the upper point hung a shiny red heart. On the crescent sat a Pierrot figure, not looking sad, not looking happy. The face questioned the onlooker in a surprised, anxious manner, and one white-gloved hand was raised as if to beckon you. In the background were shiny silver stars.

'I walk behind the science labs and it's so strange not seeing you around joking and mucking about with everyone. I feel like I expect to see you come around one of the corners at any moment. See! Your spiritual presence dwells here! I love being back at school but I miss you. It's different without you.'

Matteo was in Adelaide again and said he'd see us at Maria and Mike's. It was a hot Saturday evening and we laughed and chatted, but Matteo sensed the strain and watched me attentively.

Maria was asking Matteo about Jon. I kept my eyes on the television, trying to concentrate on the foolish pranks of a comedian. My back felt sticky with perspiration. I leaned forward, elbows on knees, so I couldn't see either of them. Matteo was explaining the problems but not what caused them. He called it lymphoma. His final sentence lunged at me. 'He's in a hospice now.'

I turned to him. 'What's a hospice?'

'I thought you knew he was there. It's like a hospital but

for the dying. He's lost the use of his legs and all bladder and bowel control. He needs full-time care and medication because he's in a lot of pain. His intestines are perforating, and he gets very swollen with infection. He wasn't this bad at the beginning of the week. The day before he went into the hospice I phoned his place in the morning. Kevin answered, and said Jon had fainted in the living-room and been there all night until he'd arrived. I tried to imagine what it must've been like waiting hour after hour for someone to show up. I went over. Kevin had to leave so I minded Jon until some nurses turned up.'

I stared at the television screen. It had blurred and senseless caricatures gyrated and mimicked the antics of human beings. I looked away to the window and the night sky. The room had blurred. I felt heat rising and a sudden sensation as if I would faint. I buried my face in my hands. Matteo put one hand on my heaving shoulder. Rob clasped my leg.

'There's nothing we can do. We've got to face it,' Matteo said. 'If you intend to go over, that's what you'll find.'

'When are you going?' Maria asked. She was kneeling in front of me.

I wiped my face and looked at her. 'Next weekend.'

Maria looked at me with concern. Her eyes questioned me. She wanted to know the truth. My eyes pleaded with her not to ask. She had asked before if Jon had AIDS and I had shaken my head. I would lie again tonight if I had to. But it might not be as convincing and it was not the end of the journey yet.

Before Matteo left, we planned to see each other in Sydney. He would meet me at the hospice.

'Let me know if you want company. I'll go with you,' Maria said.

'I'll be going by bus, and it's a long way.'

'Are you going, Rob?'

'No. I really think Maria wants to go alone.'

I smiled at Rob. He knew me well. 'Yes,' I said. 'I've done it before.'

'But it's a long way to be alone thinking about this, especially the way back.'

Maria was wonderful. I loved her so much. But how could I explain that her solid friendship would intrude on this other friendship? There was something I had to do for Jon, something he was challenging me to confront. 'I'll be all right. I'll ask for next Friday off on Monday.' We kissed each other. She would be there for me later.

Driving to work on Monday, I rehearsed my lines. They wavered between the truth and the cover. In the rear-view mirror, I composed a face. It did not need much construction. My eyes were strained, my cheeks pale.

Scene one. Peter was in his office. As I approached him, I felt like I was in a piece of film that was being replayed. I remembered a Friday afternoon when I needed to see a doctor, except it wasn't my doctor. I remembered a Monday morning I had to tell him my friend had a terminal disease except it wasn't the disease that I said it was. 'I want to ask for Friday off. Jon's not well and I want to go over this weekend. He's only got a couple of months to live.'

Peter listened, his eyes kind and understanding as usual. 'That's fine. You should let Bill know.'

Scene two. I made my way to the principal's office. I knocked on his open door. He put down his pen and asked me in, his voice crisp and refined. I sat opposite his desk and repeated my lines.

He leaned back on his chair, hands behind his head, looking silently past me to the clock. The smile had gone. 'Why the bus?'

'I can't really afford the plane fare.'

'How long did you want to be there?'

'The weekend.'

'But you'd need Friday and Monday for travelling.'

'Yes.'

He lifted his pen and tapped it loudly on his desk. He hummed a tune for a moment.

'I think we can organise for you to go by plane.' He leaned forward, looking at me intently. 'Jon is dying. I think it would be in line with the philosophy of our school if we sent you over by plane. You put in the money you were going to pay for the bus.'

'It'd be great –'

'At recess-time, I'll call a staff meeting and ask people to donate money towards the flight, and whatever is not raised will be put in by the school. It's the Christian thing to do.'

'Could you ask if people want to send over any cards or small gifts? I'll take them over.'

'You'll be our ambassador,' he agreed. 'Far more worthwhile than a wreath for the funeral.' He stood up, showing me to the door.

I was caught between emotions. The support and understanding he had shown were exhilaratingly human. And yet, I felt angry and guilty. Even as I thanked him, I wanted to shout, 'No, it's not like that at all.'

During the meeting, I sat quietly listening to the principal's steady voice and the sounds of concern and sympathy of others. My heart thumped. Why was such deception necessary?

The guilt gnawed at me. They were going to part with money, they were going to give cards and gifts which would express certain emotions and assumptions. They should know. But I had made a promise, and the truth would hold until Jon's death.

That evening I telephoned Kevin. 'How's he coping in the hospice?'

'He fluctuates. At times, he believes this is it. He says he doesn't want to lose control over what's happening to him, but he wants to hurry the journey. At other times, he's full of life and making plans for the year.'

'Do his parents know?'

'Yes, they've been told. They're coming to Sydney later

this week. You'll finally get to meet them.'

'You sound concerned.'

'They never wanted to acknowledge me, Maria. If they think they can come here and take over.' Kevin sighed. 'But we'll cross that one when we have to.'

The rest of the week was crowded with emotions. Talk of death and friendship. I was warned what to expect. Dying cancer patients look horrific, I was told. What about dying AIDS patients, I wanted to ask.

Jim and Michael asked how I felt.

'I want to see him, just to tell him how much we love him.' I looked back at the people laughing and talking. 'I feel angry,' I whispered. 'How many would really care?'

'All that doesn't matter,' Jim assured me. He gave me a hug.

Michael waited for Jim to go. He looked around. 'Tell Jon something for me. Tell Jon I really admire and respect him. Give him a big hug and kiss for me. Tell him I always wanted to do that, but I never had the courage to. I bloody wish I had.' He moved away.

'Hey!' I grabbed his arm. 'Kiss me and I'll pass it on!' He smiled awkwardly and kissed me.

24

THE FIRST TIME I've flown at night, through the engulfing darkness, is on my way to see a dying friend in Sydney. Car lights form serpents along main arteries, slithering from one destination to another without getting anywhere.

Robbo is waiting for me. I recognise the hesitant smile and warm eyes instantly. We embrace. Having no baggage to collect, we head quickly towards the car-park. As we step outside, I feel the damp sticky air. It's been raining – a steamy summer shower.

Robbo quickly lights a cigarette before he starts the engine. His fingers tremble, and the cigarette quivers between his lips. His car is old and weather-beaten, complaining loudly at having to be rushed through Sydney streets. When we talk about Jon, he becomes physically agitated, and his voice loses animation. He lights another cigarette and draws heavily on it. He clutches the steering wheel, sitting forward as he drives. He tells me what the last few days have been like in the hospice, the warmth and compassion of the staff, the homely atmosphere. He talks about Jon's last few days in his unit, to be cleaned and fed, needing to be rescuscitated after his daily fainting spells.

He has come from the hospice where Jon was sitting up in bed watching friends talking about him, smiling in response to questions and pieces of humour. I tell Robbo I'd like to see him tonight, but he tells me Kevin is still at the hospice and wants me to wait for him at their place. Kevin thinks it's better if he 'prepares' me for what I'll find and then maybe we can go. It is about half past nine now, but the hospice has no set visiting hours.

We park outside a corner pub. I step outside and see the lacework, the terraces around me and feel I am in another world. We walk to the house a few doors down. It is pleasant. The kitchen is an alcove. The backdoor steps lead down to a minuscule backyard that overlooks four neighbouring minuscule backyard gardens.

Robbo and I drink, talk, and wait for Kevin. Sven hovers around, looking older and forlorn.

About half an hour later, Kevin enters. He smiles through weary and glassy eyes, hugs me, and then sits opposite me, just watching. His fingers run through his hair now and again, particularly when he speaks. He is thin, fragile, and tension lines his face.

'So tell me,' I begin.

The words pour out, frank and calm, and weighted with sadness and love. Kevin speaks of Jon's feeling of loss of dignity, of his humiliation and mood swings. 'He says the hospice is the end of the road, and yet he wants to get better and go home. I don't know what to say to him.'

Robbo prepares two dope joints. Kevin lights his and draws in quickly. He looks at the joint. 'I hope this relaxes me enough to get some sleep, to stop me thinking.' He looks at me, almost apologetically. 'I can't fall asleep anymore without this little friend.'

Robbo smokes in silence.

'What can I do?' I ask.

'He knows you're coming. He's been looking forward to seeing you all week.' Kevin's eyes water, but the smile persists. 'When I told him on Monday night, you should've seen his smile. His eyes lit up, he almost clapped his hands like a little kid, and then he started crying.' Kevin shifts, blinking away tears as he draws on his joint. 'I think you should know this. I think you would want to know, but don't take it in a bad way. It's just poor Jonno seeing it all in some sort of pattern that we can't see. He cried, and said, "If Maria's coming, then I know I'm dying. She's coming to see me die." And he's been getting worse all week.'

The room blurs. 'Oh no, I didn't mean to –'

'No, don't take it wrong. He really wants you here. He asks about you a hundred times a day. It's like he's waiting for you.'

'When can I see him? Can we go now?'

'I think it's best not to. His old college friends and his parents have been with him all day. He was exhausted by the time they left. The sister gave him some morphine to get him to sleep. Come with me tomorrow morning. He'll be waking around seven.'

'Morphine!' Robbo rasps. His foot taps the floor urgently.

'How long has he got?' I ask.

'A few days, they think. By Wednesday. The pain is too strong. There's nothing they can do. He stopped eating

---

143

today. And his insides are all infected.' Kevin folds his arms across his chest.

I feel so cold. I wrap my arms around myself and cry.

'When are you going home?'

'I've got a flight booked for Sunday evening.'

He nods but shifts awkwardly. His eyes shine despite the film of smoke in front of them.

'But all I have to do is phone. I'll stay as long as you need me.'

'That'd be great. Help us take care of him, and talk together, you know?'

We sit in silence. When he looks at me again, his eyes are red-rimmed. The dope has cast a slight waxy finish over them. 'He looks very different. I should warn you. Very thin. Lost a lot of hair. Awful bruises. If you find it hard to be with him, that's okay. Some would say it's a ghoulish sight.'

'It?' I query. 'It's Jon. My friend. I know what he was like.'

'He's got no idea how he's looking. Hasn't seen a mirror since he went in to the hospice.'

'He always said he wanted to die with dignity.'

'He's putting up a bloody good fight.'

'What should I do while I'm with him?'

'Talk to him. Touch him. His parents are finding that hard to do. Their own fucking son!' Kevin pauses and draws on his joint. 'We've been giving him washes, you know, sponge baths. You could help if you like. Shave him, dress him. Just show we care, really. That he's our Jonno.'

After Robbo and Kevin have gone to their beds, I lie awake for hours on the lounge, listening to the sounds of traffic and dogs. 'Just show we care, really.' I have never had to confront death. 'That he's our Jonno.' Yes, he's my friend. I'm here to go with him for part of the journey and wave goodbye before he leaves.

At about one in the morning, the front door opens. I see a shadow of a tall, well-built man. A smell of aftershave fills the room. It must be Terry. He notices my figure on the lounge on his way to the kitchen but doesn't say anything. I hear him open the fridge, pour a drink, and walk past me again to the stairs. His footfalls on the stairs are heavy thuds. I hear Terry and Kevin whisper to each other. My heart aches for the old days when Jon and Kevin whispered in our spare bedroom.

Throughout the night, Sven nuzzles at the door adjoining the kitchen and lounge. He whines and snuffles in the kitchen, and then scratches at the door, wanting to come into the lounge. He paces about in the kitchen, his claws tapping on the linoleum, restless and uneasy. Why doesn't he sleep? Why don't I sleep?

I see the grey light of day through a window. Sven is still pleading, a constant reminder of where I am, why I am here. I discover I had gone to bed in my clothes as if I'd known I wouldn't sleep. I feel like I've waited all night for morning.

At about six, Kevin comes downstairs. His eyes are swollen, his face pale and lined. His newly washed hair is slicked back. He looks like a child caught in an awkward situation.

I go upstairs to the bathroom and tidy my hair and face in a makeshift way. I cannot be bothered washing my face.

Downstairs, Kevin and I prepare some orange juice, and munch on some honeydew melon as we stand on the backdoor step, looking up at the cloudy sky that sprinkles raindrops. We feel the crisp air slowly losing its freshness over the backyards and roofs of Sydney. We talk in subdued tones, in short brief phrases, and watch Sven pace about, sniffing around our legs, in and out of the house, troubled. 'He knows something's wrong,' Kevin says. Sven scratches at some plants in the garden. 'Look. My plants are dying. I've neglected them. I hope it keeps raining.'

The stillness, the sprinkling rain, the growing musty heat, the backyards of rusting iron and mouldy wood, sadden me. I wonder who lives in the adjoining houses. Kevin smiles at my question. 'Interesting types. Offbeat. Next door is a middle-aged eccentric. He lives with his mother. He hangs out his washing each evening. We rarely see the old woman, just this glimpse of pink cardigan and grey hair. Terry thinks he's retarded. I don't know. Just big and awkward. Across the road is a family, a couple of noisy kids, a screaming mother and a couple of men. One must be the father. She smothers both with kisses. The kids play on the street and are really noisy on Sunday mornings.'

25

IT'S A SHORT DRIVE to the Sacred Heart Hospice. Across the road from St Vincent's Hospital, down the road from King's Cross, a few paces down from Oxford Street. Memories flood me. The sense of a menacing Sydney scorches me.

We park outside the hospice wall. We walk through the gates, into the foyer. It looks so new, shades of blue and grey. Pleasant young nurses. They smile at Kevin. In the lift, Kevin presses the second floor button.

I feel strange. I'm looking for comforting signs in the material things about me. I make a mental note of the smiling nurses, the pink flowers on desk-tops and the pastel prints on the walls. The lighting is subdued. No stark images. Everything seems hushed, acquiescent, accepting.

The lift opens onto a foyer. On one side are glass doors leading to a balcony with white iron lacework garden chairs and tables. Flower-boxes overflow with greenery. White concrete pots hold flowering plants. This could be part of a European sidewalk cafe.

We walk down a silent corridor with wards on either side. The doors are all shut. At the end of the corridor a long cream counter appears. Nurses in white and blue sit behind it writing in books. They look up and greet us with smiles. Kevin asks about Jon. 'He's woken out of the morphine, but he's probably still groggy. The doctor was in earlier this morning because he was crying out during the night. We may have to give him more morphine when the pain becomes unbearable.' The nurse is in her late twenties, brown hair tied neatly back, eyes wide and clear. She seems calm and detached enough to be able to do what she needs to do without being crushed.

Kevin discusses the morphine doses with her. I look around. My palms are perspiring, sticking to the gifts and envelopes I'm carrying. Directly to the left of the counter, on the other side of another corridor, is an open door. My eyes look in. My heart retreats at the sight. My mind is having difficulty registering the sight of bony feet and legs curled in a foetal position, lying immobile on a bed. They belong to the safe world of films, television, textbooks and pictures of the victims of concentration camps and famine. But this is here in an Australian hospital bed. I feel helpless and angry, and wonder about the poor person, what he or she is dying from.

Kevin thanks the nurse and begins to move. I walk slightly behind him. I have a few seconds to wonder how the sight of Jon will compare to what I've seen when I realise we are walking towards that door, and stepping into that room.

It seems that the seconds have stretched, that time has gone into slow motion as my emotions and my rational thoughts struggle to acknowledge the sight. The room seems to swim, and I clench my fist, digging my fingernails into my palm, hoping that the sharp stinging will steady me. My other hand clutches the items tightly.

My eyes have slowly, painfully slowly, followed the form on the bed from the feet and legs to the baggy grey shorts, the prominent hip-bone jutting out under the material; the t-shirt clinging to a rib-cage over which a wasted arm and hand rest. The collar-bone sits just under the mottled dark skin, and the head, the skull about to split the skin, and the remaining wisps of hair. I do not recognise the face. I cannot see it. It's as if my eyes have gone out of focus, like a camera lens that has just been tampered with. I do not want to look at it. I must.

Is it Jon? Can death so emaciate a face that it takes away the semblance of the person who was once full of life? I see the angular cheek-bones, jutting jaw, thin nose, hollow temples, sallow skin, enormous dark eyelids stretched thinly over bulging eyes, dry cracked purple lips, and the gaping mouth revealing the long yellow teeth. Is it Jon?

The focus re-adjusts. Within and beyond the ugliness, the distortion, my mind sees Jon, my heart acknowledges the friend I love and the sense of revulsion abates.

Kevin calls him, briskly and cheerily. 'Wake up, Jon. Guess who's here to see you. Come on, wake up!' He has moved to the opposite side of the bed, gently shaking his shoulder. He kisses the hollow temple.

The eyes slowly open, and turn upwards. My eyes meet his. I never knew what huge, grey-blue irises he had. They seem to have enlarged, as if there is so much more to see now.

Now I know what I have come to do. This is the end-piece, the final leg of the journey. I have come to help my friend die. I have come to be given the most precious gift anyone could give me.

'It's Maria,' Kevin says.

A smile stretches the mouth into a wide grimace. A hand floats upwards towards me. Instinctively, I take it, cold and clammy, in mine. The bones threaten to disintegrate in my grip.

'Yes, it's me. So good to see you.' From inside me, my voice arrives, sounding strangely natural. I lean over and kiss his sunken cheek. My actions feel automatic, as if I've gone into automatic drive.

Jon attempts to squeeze my hands. 'Maria,' he says in a deep, throaty voice. 'You've come, then.'

'Yes! I've been wanting to for so long. To be with you.'

Jon tries to raise his head but it falls back on the cushion. Kevin helps him to sit up. He hasn't let go of my hands. As

Kevin adjusts him into a sitting position, Jon groans slightly and Kevin apologises.

He looks at me again. Kevin indicates that I should speak louder. Jon isn't hearing very well. 'I'm sending you everyone's greetings. I've got so many cards for you, and gifts and things. Look! A school annual. Everyone sends their love.'

'That's lovely. We'll look at them later.' He looks past me. It hits me that he's beyond these items of daily human existence. I sit on a chair next to the bed trying to make eye contact, but he keeps looking away into the distance. Yet, as I speak, he smiles and nods. The eyelids slowly descend over his eyes and then struggle to re-open. His fingers quiver slightly in my hands.

Kevin motions that he is going to talk to the nurse. His eyes are tearful.

I am alone with Jon, or this travesty of Jon. I want to hug him tightly. I want to cry. I want to shake him, force life into him. I want him to laugh, to tease me. But he sits still, listening to the silence of the room, looking out into the emptiness next to me, holding my hand.

Maybe if I keep talking, he'll react. 'I've got so much news, Jon. Do you want to hear it?'

'Yes.' His voice is dignified, but he's not interested.

I launch into my news, which he tolerates, smiling politely at some of my attempts at humour, as if he understands I am still firmly part of this earthly world.

I stroke his dry arm. 'I'm so glad to be here with you,' I say. He still looks just past me. The smile has receded. His eyes open and close. A silent tear appears in one eye. It hovers on the edge of his lower eyelid before slowly making its lonely journey down his sunken cheek, balancing precariously above his jawbone. He squeezes my hand.

'I'm going to stay with you now.'

He squeezes my hand again. He swallows, his Adam's apple a huge stone jerking in his throat. He attempts to clear his throat, dry retches, his body jerking forward. I hold one hand tightly and place my other hand on his forehead. With a sigh, he rests back on his pillow.

'Would you like a drink, Jon?'

'Yes, that would be lovely.' He is breathing rapidly.

I raise the straw to his mouth and place it between his dry, cracked lips. He sucks feebly, stopping now and again to rest.

'Thank you.' He settles back again.

I sit down, take his hand and caress it. I notice the gold wedding band he always wore is not on his finger. 'Where's your ring, Jon?'

He raises his hand to look at it. He frowns slightly. 'I think – in the drawer.'

I open the drawer and pick it up. I'm about to return it, realising his finger has shrunk so that the ring probably doesn't stay on, when he says, 'Give it to me.' I place it in his palm. He looks at it intently. 'Put it on my finger.'

Gently, I slide it on his ring finger. It is very loose. I slide it onto his middle finger. He gazes at it with a smile.

Kevin comes in again. Jon smiles at him, holding out his hand. 'Look, Kevin. Maria found my ring. I'm going to wear it now. It looks very lovely.'

'Yes, it does,' Kevin says steadily. He glances at me and smiles in response to my awkward shrug. 'Time for a wash, hey, Jonno?' he asks. 'A nice shave and wash will make you feel comfortable.'

Jon turns to me, holding out both hands. 'I'm going to get myself a ring on each finger later.' He seems contented with the thought. Kevin and I exchange questioning looks. Only Jon knows what he means.

I stand up, prepared to help. So gently, Kevin undresses him. With soft strokes, he sponges the skeletal body, the tautly stretched abdomen that is a purplish, mottled colour; the bruises on his back and where buttocks once were, but where now skin sags beneath the pelvic bone; the shrivelled penis attached to a catheter and a plastic bag half full of bloodied urine; the penis, functionless and powerless.

Jon's body is so light. I hold him, shifting him so Kevin can wash him. 'Hug me,' I tell Jon as Kevin rolls him towards me. With every movement, Jon groans, his forehead frowning, his mouth grimacing. 'I'm sorry, Jon. I know.' Kevin keeps saying. 'I'm trying not to hurt.' There is so much love and tenderness in the way he moves and speaks.

Kevin gently holds Jon's face in his hands. 'You look at me with that good eye, Jon, you flirt. Now, do you want a shave, handsome?' He moves his face closer to Jon's until the lips almost touch. Jon basks in the warmth. His own hand rises and touches Kevin's face. Kevin kisses his lips tenderly.

'Yes, please,' Jon whispers with pleasure.

I sit on the bed and hold Jon's hand while Kevin carefully lathers Jon's face and then painstakingly shaves him. I feel so sad, but there is much love here. I notice Kevin nicks him a couple of times as he tries to ease the razor over the bony angles of cheekbone and jawbone. I dab at the blood with cotton-wool.

After the shave, we dress him and sit him up. He seems more alert, fresher. 'Now you look so much better,' Kevin declares. I see a comb on the bedside cabinet and, gently, I run it through his wispy hair.

'I feel better, yes,' Jon says, looking from Kevin to me and back with a grateful smile.

'Fresh and clean, hey?' I say.

Jon turns to me. I sit on the bed close to him. 'Were you here last night?' he asks with concern in his voice.

I look across to Kevin. He nods rapidly. I look back at Jon, stroking his arm. 'Yes! I came in as soon as I got out of the airport.'

'Oh, good.' He seems relieved. 'We talked?'

'Lots! We talked about everything. You really made me laugh, too.' I don't seem to be able to stop lying.

'Good.' He looks to the side of me again. 'I can't say much now.'

'That's okay. Have a rest now. You can talk to me later.'

He nods and closes his eyes.

Kevin and I sit silently looking at each other, now and again glancing at Jon. A minute or two later, a tear falls from his left eye. He opens both eyes and looks just past me again. I try to meet his gaze. Somehow, he manages to avoid looking directly at me, as if the real being he wants to talk to is sitting next to me. 'Maria, are you being serious?' he asks, his voice trembling.

'What do you mean? You know me! I'm never serious, Jon. I'm a stirrer.' I chuckle awkwardly.

'Are you being serious now? I'm being serious now.' His voice sounds pained. He struggles to steady his twitching mouth, looking intently just beyond me.

'Yes, Jon. I'm very serious now. I'm here with you and I'll stay with you.' I realise ashamedly that he doesn't want facile cheering. He wants acceptance and support as he makes his way. I reach out and stroke his cheek. He closes his eyes again and leans slightly towards my hand, a gentle smile on his face. Another tear-drop winds its path down his cheek.

A sister enters the room. 'Is it time for another shot, Jon?' she asks with a crisp voice and gentle pat on his shoulder. She nods at me, and Kevin introduces me.

Jon nods.

'Do you feel a lot of pain?'

'Yes.'

'Where? Point for me.'

Jon's hand moves down to his abdomen.

'Would you like Kevin and Maria to stay while I give you the injection? I'd prefer if they left the room for a while. Do you mind if they leave the room?' I notice how she speaks to him as if he is in control, directing the moves. Kevin had spoken in a similar way.

He reflects and then responds, 'I don't mind. Whatever you would prefer, sister.'

She smiles. 'They can go for a little walk. What do you think, Jon?'

He nods.

She opens the door for us, whispering, 'Time out.'

26

KEVIN AND I walk to the far end of the corridor. There is a window overlooking the street. The sun makes my eyes squint after the soft lighting of Jon's room. The fresh air bites into my lungs. The noise of traffic and activity seem to jostle me and loosen the mask of strength I've been wearing. Kevin holds me tight as I sob, as my body trembles and Jon's body and face hover in front of my closed eyes. Kevin weeps softly, whispering, 'Let it out. Don't bottle it in.'

After a few minutes, I find my voice, muffled against his shoulder. 'I'm such a weakling.'

'No. You were very strong. I knew you would be. You have to help me keep going.' He weeps silently into my shoulder.

'I didn't think he'd look like that. You warned me –'

'It hurts to see him like that. I still find it very hard.'

'It's so unfair.'

Kevin moves away, sinks into an armchair, the sun lighting up his haggard face. He lights a cigarette. 'We can't see the fairness.' His eyes fill with tears. 'I'd like him to die with dignity and self-respect. A sense of being in control.'

'It must've been very hard for you these last few weeks.'

'It's been very hard for a long time. Someone you love, and you don't love anymore. Someone you feel so responsible for and guilty about. In the meantime, you have a great new relationship. But you still want Jon to be around, to be your lifelong friend. Instead, he's the dying ex-lover who says some bloody awful things in anger. You yell abuse back, and then you hate yourself because you know he's hitting out because he's dying. Other times, he's silent – the suffering martyr. You yell abuse at him to try to stop him feeling sorry for himself. Other times he's a conniving bastard who makes cynical comments about your new relationship, telling Terry he knows what I'm like and Terry's the fool for becoming involved.' Kevin shakes his head. 'God, I could hate him. But I love him.'

The sister approaches us. 'He's all right now. The morphine will soothe any pain. But it does keep him fairly groggy. Stay with him. He may mumble all sorts of things. He's in a half world. Sort of here and there, if you know what I mean.'

I do. He's hovering on the edge of the cliff, contemplating the plunge, but drawing back, frightened of the fall.

She pats Kevin's hand. 'Will you be all right?' She's a nun, middle-aged, plump, motherly. She could be anyone's Mum. She cares. She sees humanity in its nakedness and knows there is no hierarchy. We're all the same at the end.

'Thanks. I'm okay,' Kevin says. 'Do you know when his parents will be arriving?'

'Soon. They said by mid-morning. They would like time alone with him. I understand it's difficult for you, but they are his parents. They have their own dilemmas to face now.' She smiles and walks away.

'Parents!' Kevin stands up and moves next to me at the window. He hits his fist on the ledge. 'They've been here a week. They come here with a bible and sing hymns and pray over him and just don't see what he's going through! What kind of God do they believe in? Doesn't sound like the one my parents and I believe in. Or the God that the Sisters of Charity who run this hospice believe in.' He shakes his head. 'I know they love him. They do love him. But it's the kind of loving he could do without right now.'

'How are they treating you?'

'They try to ignore me. I'm the disgusting boy who led Jon astray. He would have grown out of this nastiness if it wasn't for me. They don't want to know me or the truth.' He leans his head on the window and weeps silently. I place one arm around his waist and rest my head on his shoulder. ' They give me just a brief smile,' he continues, 'and then they imply I should get out of the room while they try to save their son's soul.' He lights another cigarette and smokes feverishly. 'You know, they come here, touch him briefly, and then wash their hands before going.' I shake my head in disbelief.

'They're at a loss, Kevin. They don't know what to do. Isn't there anybody who can help them?'

'What about your parents? Would they know what to do?'

'I guess my parents are used to expressing their emotions. I can't imagine my parents ever being like Jon's, no matter what I'd done, no matter if they didn't understand. But then my parents see themselves as ignorant and don't pretend they know everything.' My voice is angry, loud.

Kevin smiles wistfully. 'Your parents understand what's really important to understand. So do mine. My Mum would be handing out cups of tea and buttered scones to all my visitors, crying and laughing along with them.'

'Surely they realise it's too late for their religious theory. Can't they see what it must do to Jon?'

'They don't know how to see. They've never really seen who he is. Never accepted him as gay, just as fallen by the wayside. Now they're faced with this thing on that bed.'

'They must be suffering, Kevin, knowing they will lose the son they never really got to know. Can you imagine what that must feel like? Jon always said they really loved him.'

Kevin crushes the butt of his cigarette in an ashtray. He nods.

'What about his sisters?'

'The sister in Africa is on her way here.'

'Well, we're also part of his family.'

Kevin smiles. 'Let's go to him. If you want to, that is.'

I take his arm. 'That's my friend. It's only a gruesome mask he's wearing.'

Dying is losing some of its mystery.

27

ANOTHER HOUR PASSES. Every now and again, Jon mumbles words we do not understand. We try to respond. Then he slips away. We offer him drinks, place cool towels on his forehead, wipe the perspiring palms, and stroke the thin dry arms.

I look around the room. On a high corner shelf sit some cards including my Valentine's Day card. On a side cabinet is a cassette player and some tapes. A small cupboard holds a few items of clothing. His bedside cabinet holds fruit and a drink, and a box of white tissues. On the other side of the bed is a small adjoining room with a basin and bath and shower. A sliding-door leads to a balcony that looks down on the busy street. Sun streams through the curtainless glass, brightening the grey-blue decor of the room. On the wall opposite the bed is a pastel print of Sydney Harbour with the Bridge and Opera House in prominent position. Sydney sits overseeing the scenes played out in this room.

Kevin and I talk very little. He empties the urinal bag at one point, sending a pungent smell through the room. Most of the time we sit on opposite sides of the bed, touching Jon, adjusting the sheet, staring at the minute changes occurring in him. His facial skin seems to be shrinking further, the colour becoming a deeper reddish-purple.

'He's so different today,' Kevin whispers. 'Yesterday, he was quite alert, waiting for you. He read your Valentine's Day card. Last night, I said you'd arrived and he seemed to begin slowing down, complaining about pain and asking for morphine. He's just drifting away. He's hardly said anything to you.'

'He used to say to me, "There's nothing more to be said, Maria." '

'He's been holding on waiting to see you. I think he'll die soon.'

We hear a shuffling near the door. Two old people enter the room. I stand and happen to glance at the clock. It is ten.

The woman is tall, solid, carefully dressed, grey hair neatly tied into a bun. She carries a brown handbag. Her blue eyes are sharp and piercing, darting quickly around. The man is slightly stooped, a nervous grin on his face. His hands tremble slightly. He seems to cower behind the woman, glancing at us from above her shoulder. Yet, in him, I see what Jon would look like if he could live to old age, the white thinning hair and roundish face.

I move away from the chair near Jon's bed and walk to the opposite side, standing behind Kevin who remains seated.

She nods at Kevin in greeting and with a fixed, wary smile looks expectantly at me. Kevin introduces me in a flat voice. 'This is Maria. From Adelaide. I'm sure Jon must have mentioned her to you.'

Her smile widens and becomes genuine. He smiles too, and comes forward past his wife saying, 'Yes, Jon would often write about you.'

'You've had a child,' she says, taking up the story. 'Jon read us a letter you wrote to him about that. I hope she's well. And your husband too.' She is pleasant and kind.

I fit their image of a suitable friend. Married, maternal, expounding the joys of both conventions in a long letter to their son. And from Adelaide, city of churches. I smile, but anger boils inside me. Deep down, I feel a surge of love for Jon. He used my letter to get through to them.

The mother takes the chair I've vacated. The father hovers next to her, hands in pockets. She kisses Jon briefly on the forehead, and then sits back holding his hand. 'Jonathon. Jonathon. Mother's here. And father's here too.' The old man's lips tremble.

Jon stirs and turns slightly towards her.

'Yes, it's mother and father, Jonathon.'

'Mother,' he mumbles.

'Yes. Mother loves you very much.' She begins to cry and bites her lower lip. The father closes his eyes tightly and grasps his wife's shoulder for support. I want to tell them that it's all right to cry.

She regains her composure and pats her husband's hand while holding Jon's. 'We have always loved you. You know that, don't you, Jonathon? We've always prayed for you, dear.'

A tear appears at the corner of Jon's eye and makes its way down as he nods slowly. Then he turns his head away from them.

'Yes, we'll let you sleep,' she says, releasing his hand. 'You sleep peacefully, dear.' She looks up at us.

'He's had morphine injections for the pain,' Kevin tells them. 'So he's groggy.' She doesn't respond. He continues. 'He hasn't got long.'

Before Jon's parents have to deal with this, Robbo arrives. He takes one look at the parents, nods curtly at them, and walks out again after a concerned look at Jon. Kevin stands up and silently follows. The eyes of both parents follow him.

Awkwardly, I make to move out. 'There's no need for you to go, dear,' she says sweetly. 'We know how much you meant to Jon.'

So many beginnings of sentences get caught in my throat. He loved Kevin more than he loved me. Kevin and Robbo have done so much for him. Why is it only acceptable for me to stay with you? Those two are just like me. We all love your son.

I smile weakly, clenching my fits to keep my fury under control. I sit on the arm of the chair, waiting for an opportune moment to present itself. The mother is fussing with the bed linen. The father begins to roam about the room. He picks up some of the cards and reads them. 'They're from people at work,' I say.

'They express some very lovely sentiments.' He looks so sad.

'They absolutely adored Jon at work. He was a great

teacher, a great friend.' Have you ever thought about that, I want to add.

The mother looks up from the bed. 'We have never really known much about Jon's teaching career.'

'He was an excellent teacher. Kids loved him.'

The father picks up the copy of the 1988 school annual. 'They sent it to Jon to show him the valete message,' I explain. He turns a few pages and then finds the piece Michael had written about Jon.

I see the old man's lower lip tremble uncontrollably. He clutches the annual to his chest and sobs. His wife rises to comfort him. 'You mustn't upset yourself so. It's not good for you. Control yourself, please.'

He hands her the annual. 'Read it. It's beautiful.'

She returns to her seat, reading the article. At the end, tears fall silently. She looks back at her son as if she's seeing him in a new light and takes his hand again.

'Did so many people really care for him?' she asks.

'Oh, yes. He gave so much to everyone. He was a decent human being. A real Christian.' Do I sound too insistent? They must know. I swallow before the words tumble out. 'You should be very proud of your son.'

She bows her head. Her husband stands next to her. They weep together. Now and again, he shakes his head. My heart goes out to them, even as I want to shout at them in rage.

I walk quietly out of the room. They need to be alone with their son, and their grief and regrets.

Kevin and Robbo are sitting near the counter. 'What's going on?' Kevin asks.

I sit down next to him. 'They read the piece in the school annual. I think they're facing the fact that they never gave him the credit he deserved, and that must be a very painful thing for parents.'

Twenty minutes later, Kevin asks the sister if she could go in and 'check'. As the door swings open, we see Jon's father standing at the foot of the bed, one hand over his eyes. The sister pretends to check the urinal bag and then walks out, shutting the door behind her. 'The mother's praying very softly and holding his hand.' She places her hand on Kevin's arm 'Try to understand. It's what they know. But they do seem closer to him today.'

28

GARY AND LINDA arrive with their baby son, and we sit in the foyer and talk about Jon and his parents. 'They're old,' Gary says, a methodical, logical person. 'They're from a different world. I remember when we were kids – they've always been set in their ways. So many of our parents were.'

They go into Jon's room, leaving the door open behind them. The greetings and pleasantries gush from Jon's parents. Linda gives the mother the baby to hold. The father moves to the door and shuts it.

Kevin and Robbo look at each other. 'Time for lunch,' Robbo says dryly. I decide not to go with them. Matteo may be arriving soon. They promise to bring me back some chocolate and milk.

I sit alone until I hear Linda's baby begin to cry restlessly and she comes out of the room, sits next to me, and gives him a bottle of milk. I've always liked her. We talk softly, about babies and motherhood, about the rude awakenings of birth and parenthood. We talk about the joy and fun of babies and our hopes for their futures. We whisper about Jon's mother and her relationship with her son.

'She must've felt this way,' I reflect. 'Jon must've been her little baby once. She must've planned to do the best for him, always be by his side. I don't understand.'

'I'm sure she did,' Linda responds, rocking her baby to sleep in her lap. 'But in a different setting.' She looks down at her son lovingly. 'You know, yesterday she asked me whether it was a good idea to take a baby into Jon's room. And when Jon held him and kissed him, she looked so uncomfortable.' Linda smiles. 'Today, she didn't say anything.' She looks directly at me. 'What a good idea bringing that school album. Jon's Dad read it out to us. He can't get over it.'

The words of the letters he had written to me in 1988 come to life as I climb the stairs to his cosy unit in the afternoon. As Kevin and Jenny, an old college friend of Jon's, collect files and personal papers, leaving only legal documents behind, I wander about, touching objects, feeling the ache inside me as I imagine Jon's last few months here.

The unit has Jon's presence in it still: it's a powerful feeling, as if he has not quite left. The shiny piano, the black Chesterfield lounge, the Swiss cuckoo clock, the photographs of European holidays with a healthier Jon smiling confidently into the camera; the photos of Kevin on a beach silhouetted against a warm orange sunset; the prints of Adonis-like, lithe males; the green well-tended plants; the Tasmanian Oak kitchen minus the vast collection of spices and herbs he once had in Adelaide; the clean bathroom and neat bedroom that provide no hint of the night-time agonies.

I picture Jon alone in this unit, finding the resilience and resoluteness in himself to leave for the hospice, for the end. Before we carry Jon's files and papers downstairs, I whisper goodbye.

Back at the hospice, the afternoon wears on. Jon mumbles now and again, groaning if he's moved. He requests sips of water. His urine is becoming more bloodied, light red in colour. His skin is drying, stretching tautly against his bones.

Kevin has been speaking to the sister. He comes into the room and puts a gentle hand on Jon's forehead. He looks troubled. 'They think he'll die tonight.'

Robbo and I sit in heavy silence.

As the afternoon unfolds, we take small breaks out on the main balcony near the lift to munch chocolate bars, breathe in fresh, warm air, and watch ordinary life continue on the road below us. By half past four, Jon seems to be more alert. Kevin and I hold his hands, offering him drinks, cooling his face and neck with a damp cloth. 'Pain,' he mutters.

'The nurse will give you more morphine, Jon. It won't be long,' Kevin says soothingly.

A few minutes later. 'The unit. Home.'

'Maria and I went there earlier. Everything's all right.'

'It's a beautiful unit, Jon. Just like you described in your letters. You've really organised it well.'

A smile quivers on his dry lips. 'I'm proud of it. You come over for lunch one day.'

'I'd love to.'

'When you're better, Jon,' Kevin adds.

'I'll be better tomorrow. No more pain tomorrow. Right, Maria?'

'No more pain, Jon. You're a survivor. I've always said that.'

'A survivor,' he repeats and closes his eyes.

Kevin whispers in my ear, 'You see? He still tries to fight it.'

'Kevin,' Jon calls, opening his eyes. Kevin sits on the bed, taking his hand and stroking his face with the other. 'I've been thinking. I'm scared. What's going to happen?' He clutches Kevin's hands in his. 'What about us, Kevin?'

As Kevin struggles for words, the sister enters to administer more morphine. This time we remain in the room. Jon lapses into a dazed silence. Kevin buries his face in his hands. I reach across and touch his shoulder. He looks up and grasps my hand.

Robbo enters with a middle-aged gentleman with large round brown eyes. He seems very serene, mystical. Robbo introduces him as the minister Jon had requested yesterday. We leave the room.

About fifteen minutes later, the minister comes out, closing the door behind him. 'He's doing well,' he says mysteriously. 'He's getting there but doesn't really want to let go yet. Help him.'

He leaves with Robbo.

At about six, Matteo walks in looking fresh in shorts and singlet. He greets Jon, kisses him and holds his hand, lips pressed tightly together, a frown marring his healthy radiance. Jon smiles briefly at him.

'What have you eaten today?' he asks me as he crushes me in a warm hug. 'You look so pale.'

'Chocolate. But I'm not hungry.'

Matteo's eyebrows rise dramatically. 'Well, you're coming with me. I'll cook you a lovely Italian dish. You need it.'

'Thanks, but I want to stay here.'

'You'll faint if you don't eat, and what good will you be then? Just an hour. You need some fresh air.'

'Go on,' says Kevin. 'I'll be here and Robbo will be back soon.'

We walk outside into the sunshine. Matteo puts a secure arm around my waist. We walk to his apartment on Rosebank Avenue. I watch the people on the sidewalks, or driving past, and note the grimness in their expressions. Matteo asks me questions and I allow myself to cry. It feels right to be crying on Sydney's streets. In Adelaide, I would be embarrassed and wipe my tears away. Here the burdens are exposed: no one pretends to smile and no one forgets the realities unless they are blinkered by alcohol and drugs.

Up on the seventh floor is a roomy, bachelor's apartment. Matteo introduces me to one of his flatmates, a creamy-skinned, clean-cut man who also comes from Adelaide, and who explains he's only wearing his underpants because he's doing the washing. He jokes that not many women have seen him in such a state. I should consider myself privileged. I laugh.

While Matteo prepares dinner, I walk out on his balcony. I

see the view but I also see the rusting rooftops, the littered alleys, the cluttered vacant lots surrounding this apartment building. I reflect that I'm tired because the view makes me dizzy. I go back to the kitchen and watch Matteo expertly prepare the meal. We talk about life and death, plans and developments, Jon's place in our lives.

Just before dinner, the other flatmate enters, a tall, muscular man with flowing curly hair and such a gentle manner. He informs me he's been 'married' to the other guy for years.

Over dinner, conversation seems to change direction freely. We talk of our childhoods, homosexuality, women, marriage, AIDS, love, ambitions. I feel rather strange sitting down to an aromatic dish of pasta discussing issues objectively and with humour while in a hospital bed only a fifteen-minute walk away, my great friend is dying. For all that, the conversation and food have cleared the heaviness. Outside that hospice, life continues, and AIDS is just a topic of sombre conversation.

Feeling refreshed, I walk back to the hospice with Matteo. It's a hot evening and the sky threatens rain. Matteo leaves me near the hospice. He must rush back home to get changed. He's going out with a 'new man'. He must iron his shirt and shave and put some wine on ice. He'll visit Jon tomorrow afternoon and stay with me there. Jon will probably have died by then, I tell him.

Matteo looks at me apologetically. 'Don't think me such a heartless person,' he pleads. 'I find it very frightening being with him. He's suffering so much, and whenever I've gone to visit, his parents or Kevin are there. I feel like an intruder. I've done what I can for Jon. I've said my goodbye. He'd understand. The last moments are for his family, Kevin and you.'

We embrace. His eyes shine. 'You go in there for me because you'll be a lot more help than I could be.' He kisses me before we head off in opposite directions.

By the time I'm back in Jon's room, the weight of what is happening hits me again. As soon as I see him I sit down and helplessly hold his hand. A sister is about to leave the room as I enter. 'Sister has asked that someone be with Jon throughout the night. It may be his last few hours,' Kevin tells me.

'He shouldn't be alone,' she says. 'Too many people die alone. That's the most dismal death.'

'I'll stay,' I tell Kevin. I don't know how I'll get through, I feel like adding, but it's something I must do.

'I'll stay as well,' says Robbo.

Kevin smiles at us gratefully. 'If anything should happen, call me. I've got to see Terry. It's just that Terry – .' His voice drifts away.

We give Jon another sponge-bath. The urine must be pure blood now. The sores are breaking. The abdomen is as hard as a rock.

29

JON HOLDS HIS FINAL Saturday night 'gathering'. Although he lies for most of the time without responding, his presence is the catalyst for laughter and companionship. Friends come in to see him, bringing fruit and chocolates, and a sense of sanity and unity. We fill the room and the adjoining corridor and the nurses smile as they walk by. We talk about Jon, about what he has meant to us, about the good times in the past. We laugh uproariously at anecdotes and reminiscences. We shed tears as the sense of impending loss descends upon us. Our moods swing wildly and we express ourselves freely. We eat fruit and chocolates, discuss babies, politics, travel and movies.

The atmosphere in the room is alive with love. Every

person feels connected with every other, and all the while, the host lies with eyes closed, now and then mumbling in response to a question, now and then casting his eyes over us with a weak smile.

I observe the people around me. I can understand why they are friends of Jon. College friends, gay friends, parents and singles; they all seem alive with the same openness and understanding.

They ask me questions. They readily admit I was often mentioned to them by Jon as 'Maria, my Italian friend'. They are interested in my background, admitting they don't know much about 'ethnic people', and ask how I came to be friends with Jon.

Someone notes how Jon's skin is drying, how it feels crinkly and brittle to the touch. Another produces hand and body lotion from a handbag. It is passed around and suddenly a warm orgy of massage is underway. We each take a limb or part of Jon's torso and begin to gently massage cream into it. We laugh and agree that Jon knows 'how to go', that he's staging his final piece for all of us to remember. At times he bestows a small smile on us and we respond in delight. He can feel the fingers, the soothing touches.

The sister looks in with eyebrows high and a wide smile at the sixteen hands gently caressing and stroking the still form on the bed. The orgiastic pleasure is met by the powerful feeling of unity and devotion. The room seems to vibrate with our rhythmic strokes and sensuality. We agree we wish we could caress away the pain and the death. Yet, we're content in knowing we are communicating to Jon's spirit our love and dedication to him.

When the parents arrive, they stop abruptly at the door, looking disconcerted. The atmosphere has been broken. The massaging gradually ceases. The lotion is put away.

The parents greet everyone and, dutifully, the guests begin to drift out of the room, but not before Jon's father has brandished the school annual, pointing to the article and imploring them to read it. They smile passively in response. What they read is nothing new to them.

Outside on the main balcony, in the musty moist night air, as the Saturday night traffic roars by, I listen to the various stories about growing up with Jon. They remember their shyness with his parents. They talk of the effects of their religion, and those who are still believers talk about the more rational modern church compared to the fundamentalism of many of their parents. So I learn that there are differences within their faith as within all others, and that I must prevent myself from stereotyping them.

Our hands still smell sweetly of the lotion. The perfume mingles with the damp hot air and provides an aura of warmth, of Jon's spirit around us. The sky is darkly clouded. After some time, the sound of traffic squishing on the wet road subsides into an insignificant hum. Lotioned hands are raised to nostrils by some as if hanging on to Jon.

After about an hour, the sister on night duty comes out to the balcony. 'Jon's parents have been told. They're quite distressed. They're going to stay the night in a room down the corridor.'

Friends exchange glances, and then look at Kevin for direction. Kevin nods and looks at Robbo and me. 'We're staying in his room,' Robbo says.

We make our way back to the room. The smell of lotion has dissipated. The parents are gone. Jon lies still, his mouth open, his breath rattling in his throat. Friends begin to make farewells, touching him gently, kissing him lightly, whispering words of love and gratitude softly near his ear. They embrace us and allow a final few tears to fall. Their final backward glances as they leave confirm their acceptance that they will not see Jon alive again.

30

IT'S NEARLY MIDNIGHT. Kevin, Robbo and I sit in the room vibrating with Jon's rattling breath, in the dimmed light of the fluro over Jon's bedhead. We sense a vacuum left by farewelling friends.

Jon's parents enter. They look weary and confused. The mother's fingers are clasped together like string. The father leans against the door, heavy with pain. The mother speaks to us, all the while staring at her son. 'You'll call us if something happens. Father here has a weak heart and needs his rest. But we will be down the corridor.' She leans forward and gently touches Jon's forehead with her fingertips. There is a gentleness and understanding in her manner. I begin to think that I've been too harsh on them. She moves back to the door and takes her husband's hand. He smiles at us tearfully. About to leave, she turns around and her eyes skim awkwardly over us. 'We thank you for staying.' They hurry out, heads bowed.

'She thanked us,' Robbo says incredulously.

We sit back in our chairs, surrounded by the rattling sound. Just before Kevin leaves, the night sister enters, and gives Jon more morphine. Almost instantly, Jon's breathing slows. As he draws in air through his open mouth, there is a deep guttural sound as if the breath is being sucked into a huge bottomless cavern. The sound is ominous and chilling. We call the sister. She holds his hands and listens. 'It's worse for you than for him. The morphine is slowing down his breathing and his whole system.'

'But is he in pain?' Kevin asks.

'Yes. There is some pain, but it sounds much worse than it is.'

The sound is upsetting Kevin. It has brought Death into the room. It is breathing voraciously, waiting to claim its next victim, pacing about the room as Jon's breathing seems to echo from the walls and ceiling. Kevin's hands shake as he gently strokes Jon's face, lips softly kissing him. He rises to leave. 'Phone if anything happens. I'll come back.' He leaves, the tears falling down his cheeks.

Robbo and I look at each other in the dimly lit room. We decide to take it in turns to get some sleep on a chair. Robbo insists I rest first. After twenty minutes or so, the rattling breath is actually beginning to lull me to sleep. My mind has found a way of temporarily escaping the confines of the room; a small knothole through which the sound of death eases into a background rhythmic drone.

Suddenly, the door opens and in rushes a night nurse. She is small, dark, with fuzzy curly hair. Her eyes are concerned. She looks Italian or Greek. 'Oh, I'm sorry. I thought Jon might be alone.'

She moves towards him and touches his face. 'We spent quite a few hours together last night, didn't we, sweetheart?' Her voice is soft and deep, slightly accented. She seems sleepy.

'We're staying tonight. He might not live long,' Robbo tells her.

She nods. 'I know. It's almost over for him.' She smiles understandingly at Robbo. She turns to me. Our eyes meet and our smiles are those of connection. We seem to know each other and, for the rest of the night and morning, we communicate to each other as much with our expressions and gestures as with our voices. 'The desk is just out here. The sister will be there. And I'll be around the patients on this floor all night. So let me know if you want something – coffee, food, a break. I'll fix a bed if you like.'

We nod and thank her. She smiles again before she leaves. 'I'm glad he's got friends with him. But it can be very difficult. We're just out here.' She points to the counter in the light-filled foyer, and the quiet movements and voices of two night sisters. As she closes the door behind her, it seems that the foyer is another world that we can see, we can pick up wafts of its calming breezes, but we're not ready to be a part of it yet.

Robbo and I sit on chairs on opposite sides of the bed.

169

Now and again, we sponge Jon's face or dampen his lips. Most of the time, we hold his hands, stroke his arms. I rest my head on his hand which lies motionless on the bed, and think. I feel numb. But sleep doesn't accompany this numbness. I seem to be waiting for something, and I keep my emotions at bay ready for the something to unleash itself.

It's hard to believe we are here, like this, in a room, severed from the Saturday night and early Sunday morning world just outside.

31

SOMETHING DESCENDS INTO the emotional silence. It is just after one in the morning. Jon's hand begins to jerk, subtly at first and then knocking against me. I look up at him, releasing his hand. Arms flail about as if he is drowning, frightened eyes flicker open and closed, teeth loudly knock each other as if an icy chill has entered his form. His whole body is being lifted off the bed in violent spasms.

Robbo places a hand firmly on Jon's shoulders to prevent the body shaking and with the other arm he encircles Jon's head, hugging it to himself, to stop the knocking and subvert the panic. I clutch both of Jon's hands and struggle to prevent them from swinging away. His fingers close tightly around my own, crushing, hanging on.

I know that need. I remember the pain of giving birth, the panic of the pain, and the need to crush Rob's hands in order to keep a hold on my sanity and life around me.

I look into Jon's face. This is the panic of dying. His emaciated face is distorted by terror and agony. The eyes want to leap from their sockets as if forced to view something they would prefer not to see and yet they must force themselves to see in order to make it invisible. The mouth grimaces in despair. His fingernails dig into my palms.

Slowly, the fit subsides. The grip on my hands eases and the heaving in the body stops. The spasmodic, guttural breathing returns to its regularity. A tear rolls out of an eye. A trickle of blood, black in the dim light, winds its way down the side of his mouth. He has bitten his tongue. But he has won the first round.

Robbo is shaking. From deep inside me, I feel fear frothing upwards, panic boiling. It's as if the spasm has been transferred to me and I suddenly feel that if I don't get out of the room for a second and hurl myself into the controlled world of the night-nurses, I'll become hysterical.

'The nurse,' I manage to gasp and wrench open the door. I move forward with long strides and slam my body into the counter. My heart pounds against my ribs. I clutch the counter for I feel I'm going to fall.

There is no one there. Oh God, I pray as I feel the panic rise again. Where is the safe world? Has death and its insurmountable reality hidden it, erased the facades that cage in the fury and despair of dying, of watching a loved friend struggle against the undefeatable opponent?

The sister appears from another ward. With relief, I try to explain. She takes my arm and we go back into the room. I sit in the chair as she takes Jon's pulse, examines his tongue, and lifts heavy eyelids. 'Call me as soon as it happens again so I can see what's going on. I need to attend to another patient down the hall. Are you two all right?'

We nod. Yet we sit on the edge of our chairs, not speaking, just straining our ears to detect the slightest change in Jon's breathing; our clammy hands sensitised to any movement in Jon's fingers. Twenty minutes later, when the second round is fought, the sister is not there, but I cannot leave Jon to get her. He needs to hold on, to crush my hands.

When he is back in his trance-like state and Robbo is wiping away more trickles of blood, I go to the door and ask her to come in. The Italian nurse also enters. This time they sit with us and wait. No one speaks. We wait for Death to try again.

In another twenty minutes, the fight is on. The sister helps Robbo hold Jon's body while the nurse keeps his mouth open to stop his teeth from tearing into his tongue. I hold his hands together.

When it's over, they look sad and gently monitor his heart rate, sponge his face, neck and hands. 'His body's systems are starting to collapse,' the sister tells us. 'These spasms are going to wear away his heart. You see, the heart of an AIDS patient is not affected. So while the rest of him is dysfunctional, the heart is still beating, carrying on.' She shakes her head incredulously. 'Inside that dysfunctioning body beats the heart of the strong thirty-one year-old man Jon was meant to be. It won't surrender easily. AIDS can bring on one of the worst deaths.' She turns to us. 'Reassure him. Help him through. If you can. If not, we will stay. He hasn't got long but he, or his heart, may be trying to prolong it. Talk to him when it happens. I think he's quite aware during those fits.'

So that is the battle. Death cannot claim him until the heart, the richest and most enduring receptacle of the body, has yielded. And yield it must, for it has lost all its allies within Jon's physical form. But it will fight on alone, the way Jon had always fought, his emotional centre refusing to lie down at death's feet.

I respect his inner strength, his insistence on surviving, on clinging to the final sensations of life.

I telephone Kevin. He arrives in fifteen minutes, looking strained and anguished. The sister enfolds him in her arms and explains the situation to him. He witnesses another fit with us and through tears asks for more morphine to be administered. The sister leaves the room to telephone the doctor.

Kevin hugs Jon's head. 'Poor Jonno. We love you. We'll take care of you. You hang on to us.'

Another battle in ten minutes and despite Kevin's efforts to keep Jon's mouth open, he has bitten his tongue again. We now talk to Jon as he struggles. We reassure him with our love. And once the breathing has become regular, we sit back and weep for his pain, for his fear and his refusal to surrender.

The sister gives him a little more morphine to reduce the fits, but they continue.

At about three o'clock, after another onslaught, Jon begins to mumble. We wet his lips with the sponge and move closer to hear him. 'Thank you,' a soft wispy voice drifts out to us from inside.

We feel our hearts being stretched and tears well in our eyes. 'Just for a sip of water? You don't need to thank us, Jonno,' Kevin tries to say lightly.

'Thank you for –' and his voice fades away. We bury our faces in his shoulders and hands, wetting his body.

At the end of another clash, Jon mutters, 'This is ridiculous.' Before the next one he tries to communicate to us. Most of the time, we can't understand what he says for the words are lost in the air but we manage to pick up 'No more' and 'Home' and again, 'This is ridiculous.'

'He's aware of what's happening,' Kevin whispers. 'I wish he wasn't.'

Robbo wanders out onto the little balcony. He smokes furiously and in a choking voice, as he looks out into the dark sky, shouts, 'If only I had some heroin with me. I'd put a stop to this. Why can't they stop this?'

Kevin rushes out to him and holds him closely, saying, 'Maybe he wants to end it himself in his way.'

But Jon is preparing for another battle, and we take our accustomed positions. We feel we are soldiers fighting alongside our brave general.

The fits are now closer together. They are exhausting us. The sister enters at around four and informs us Jon's mother has wandered down the corridor, stopped at the door and listened to Jon's breathing before silently returning to her room. Kevin does not want to tell her what is happening. The sister agrees. Robbo asks for more morphine or Valium.

After witnessing two more fits, one soon after the other, she goes to get some Valium. 'You must begin asking him to let go. He is fighting death and hurting himself. He should have died by now, but he is preventing his body from letting go. Valium will ease the pain but also dangerously slow down his breathing. I cannot administer anything more or I will have killed him. He must stop resisting and die when he is ready.'

'Maybe he isn't ready. He has a strong will,' I say.

She looks at me with a gentle smile. 'Yes, he's very strong isn't he? But his strength is hurting him. Death is the release he really needs now. He must relax and give in to it. He cannot come back to us.'

32

DEATH'S ONSLAUGHTS are plummeting into Jon's body every few minutes. We plead with him to let go, to say goodbye. I ask God to show Jon the way out.

After a siege has momentarily subsided, Jon's breathing does not return and our own breathing is suspended. Is he dead? And then, as if sucked from the deepest recesses of his lungs, a breath is swallowed in, distending his rib-cage, and then expelled with force. After each fit, the breathing becomes harder to restore, but we hear Jon struggling to draw in another breath.

The three of us are shattered. Our emotions are see-sawing in response to Jon's battles. As the fit plays out its battle between Death and Jon, we gather our strength to help him through. Once there is no breathing after the fit, we prepare to accept his death and whisper our love and farewells. And as the breath is pulled in, we feel relief and anguish that he and we must go through so much pain all over again.

Kevin's face is drawn. Robbo buries his head on Jon's shoulder, I clutch his hands. Kevin leans close to him and talks to him between the tears. 'You're so strong aren't you, Jon? You've always fought things. You won't stop fighting, even now. You're going to control this to the end and bloody well take us with you, aren't you?' He leans against Jon's temple and sobs quietly.

I find myself saying what I never thought I would ever say. I am asking my friend to die. 'Let go, Jon. Complete your journey. It hurts us so much to see you in so much pain. You know you'll always be a part of our lives. You've done enough now. Let go. Find your place out there.'

Kevin lifts his head and speaks to him again. 'Jon, listen to me. Please listen. You've got to go. You can't come back to us. We would love you to but you can't. Please relax and let it be. We love you.'

Another heart-wrenching fit. The breathing takes longer to return. But it's restored, this time with a loud sad groan. His eyeballs roll backward and the whites of his eyes shine in the dim light. Robbo begins to administer drops in his eyes.

Jon's breaths are now long sorrowful sighs. There are no more battles. A cease-fire has been called, awaiting the official announcement of the victor. We notice his feet and finger-tips are turning a mottled reddish-blue. They feel cold and lifeless.

I stroke his right hand. I turn it over and gently touch the purplish fingertips. There, in his palm, are the lines he read. I trace them with a finger, smoothing out the trials of his life. Very slowly, I trace his life-line and pause at the end. Softly, I kiss the spot where Life and Death's battles for supremacy over this body will cease. I use my finger-nail to etch an extension into the line. It is of no use.

Something makes me look up. The luminous dawn is painting the sky. I step out on the balcony and feel strangely bathed in the dawn light. The streets are empty and silent.

Everything is unusually still and peaceful. All I hear are the sighing breaths of Jon.

I continue standing there, transfixed by the silent beauty of Sydney at five-thirty on a Sunday morning in summer. There is no more rain but a sweet coolness that sends a strange tranquility into me.

I return to my chair, hold his hand again, and resting my head in his palm, fall asleep.

33

AT ABOUT SIX O'CLOCK, something rouses me. Robbo and Kevin are looking intently at Jon. There is a beautiful luminous atmosphere in the room. The sky outside has lightened further. Jon's breathing is very soft and shallow like that of a small bird.

'You're here, aren't you Jon? But not quite in your body anymore,' Kevin whispers. Later, we inform each other that we all had the distinct feeling at that moment that he was in the room, surrounding us, gently touching our souls, drifting in and out of his body, contemplating the final tearing of the threads that still bound him to life.

The eyes are still rolled back. The feet and hands are steadily turning blue and feel very cold. I can no longer clearly see the lines in the palms for they seem to have swollen with collecting blood.

Kevin breaks the penetrating silence. 'Jon. You look so sad now. Why do you look so sad?' The face has settled into a look of misery, of resignation. Some sort of decision has been made.

I feel cold fingers move gently beneath my hand.

Suddenly, the hand jerks up and sweeps across to Kevin in a familiar, caressing gesture.

Jon's eyes roll back into focus and he looks at each of us.

His face radiates joy, his mouth gives a smile of pure delight. His look of absolutely pure rapture seems to lift us and we find ourselves standing, smiling with him, trying to talk to him.

What is happening? Something wonderful is happening.

And then we imprint Jon's final smile and joyful eyes into our minds and hearts for the rest of our lives.

We say goodbye. We tell him we love him. We ask him to stay with us always.

There is no more breathing.

Jon's eyes are open. He has seen what he was waiting to see before he would let go. He has found his destination.

He looks peaceful. His smile of wonder and bliss and the confirmation of his expectations is his last lesson.

It is 6:15 am on a Sunday morning in Sydney, twelfth of February.

I look down. I am holding Jon's right hand, my palm against his.

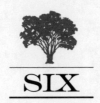

SIX

. . . a sort of cutting taken from one person and grafted on to the heart of another continues to carry on its existence even when the person from whom it had been detached has perished.

Marcel Proust

34

FROM THE MOMENT I step off the bus, on a warm January morning eleven months after Jon's death, I feel welcome.

I say goodbye to the young woman with whom I had shared a bus-seat. She sweeps her red hair out of her eyes. 'You have a good stay, you hear?' She holds out her hand and grins.

Just as I step onto the footpath, put my suitcase on the pavement, and begin to wonder whether I should try to hail a taxi or go back into the station and book one, a bright red taxi pulls up.

A cheerful driver gets out, picks up my suitcase and puts it carefully in the boot. 'Welcome to Sydney, miss!'

'Thank you, but you've already got a customer.' I point to the young bearded man sitting patiently in the front.

'Oh, it's his idea.'

'Welcome to Sydney!' the man in the front says as I sit down.

Soon, the taxi pulls up at another kerb. 'Have a marvellous time,' he says as he gets out.

I thank him. I'm beginning to wonder whether this whole thing has been planned. And when he pulls out several crumpled notes, pays for his fare, and then asks the driver to put the rest of the money towards mine, I stare in amazement, and stumble over my thanks. 'Midsummer madness!' he says and gives me a mysterious wink.

The driver chats on about his city. I mumble responses, but I'm only half listening. I'm looking through the window. The buildings seem to shimmer in the sun, and stretch out to each other.

'I think I'm going to Sydney this school holiday,' I had said to Rob before Christmas. He had smiled and replied,' I was wondering when you'd go back.'

On Saturday afternoon, I go out on my own.

I step through the gates, pass the pink and grey reception area. I take the lift to the second floor and walk down the corridor to the counter. No nurses are about. I hear people around me. The sounds are coming from the wards, but they seem to be filtering in from far away.

I walk towards the room. The door is open, the bed dishevelled. A pair of jeans hangs over the chair. The room is empty.

Jon had only been dead for a few minutes. We had cried but inside we had felt exquisite joy, relief.

Kevin looked at the body on the bed. 'He's found peace. He saw something and tried to tell us.'

The body on the bed was a decaying piece of matter that we could look at without further emotional despair. Jon's spirit was alive in the room.

We called the sister, who came in and sat down with us. 'He must've been wonderful to have so many friends. I often wish I could meet these people before they actually come to us. For when we see them, we see only the "shells". 'She stood up. 'You've been admirable. And I think Jon's parents will think so too. It's time to tell them. Be compassionate. I think they're just beginning to understand.'

We walked out of the room to a nearby office to make telephone calls. Leaving the room in the daylight was like leaving behind a wasteland after a war.

As we returned to the room, Jon's mother was coming out, face mottled and strained. Fighting back tears, she walked resolutely toward us. 'Thank you for what you did for my son.' Her trembling hand extended towards us.

'He deserved much more,' I said.

She nodded, biting her lower lip, screwing up her eyes. 'I'm just realising how proud we should be of him. Should've been.' She burst into tears and struggled to control herself. 'Father would like a few minutes. In there with Jonathon. By himself.'

She shuffled away, an old woman shattered by a new disease and whatever regrets confronted her. I wanted to call her back, to hug her and apologise for my insensitivity to their pain.

We did not enter the room until the father had come stumbling out, head bowed low. The nurse asked us if we wanted to help her prepare the body. I found myself busy in a task I had always imagined would be horrible.

Jon was in the room. I felt that strongly enough that I could calmly manouevre the torso, help bandage the jawbone to the face, weigh down the eyelids over his eyes. The body, still warm and very light, moved like a rag doll. And all the while, I felt Jon watching me, laughing at the 'obnoxious flesh' he had left behind.

I recognised the clothing, worn by a lively friend and teacher. Now, the clothes were arranged on a discoloured dummy.

The nurse draped a white cloth on a little table, with a bunch of flowers and a single white candle that threw a still glow in the room.

The sister walked in and assessed the display. She nodded her approval, adjusted a shoelace, touched the clasped hands. 'If anyone would like to see him, they will have to do so this morning. Later, he'll be put in plastic and taken down to the morgue. No one's allowed to see him after that.' She shook our hands and left.

The nurse smiled, wished us well, and walked out.

Kevin, Robbo and I were left standing silently in the room. There was a dull ache inside, a feeling of exhaustion, of peaceful resignation. It was like standing on the edge of the stage at the end of a performance, the props neatly re-arranged: Sydney's cityscape; the bowl of ageing fruit and left-over chocolates; my Valentine Card; the balcony that gave us tranquility through the night; the eye-drops; the cup of water and bent straw; the damp sponge; the cards and gifts from Adelaide; the school annual.

And the body. Neatly arranged on a smooth bed, two hands clasped together. The lines on his palms could peer at each other in the cold darkness and nod with approval. It was done. Except that he did not die alone. He hadn't lost everything.

We closed the door and thanked everyone at the desk, took the lift down and walked out through the glass doors. The mellow Sunday morning flooded us. The footpath was shiny in its clean wetness, hints of an early morning summer shower.

We stood still outside the gates of the hospice, breathed deeply and smiled at the blue sky. 'Such a beautiful morning!' Kevin shouted. 'Thank you, Jonno,' he whispered.

We looked at each other and huddled together, knowing we had shared an awesome secret, travelled a difficult road.

'May I help you?'

A young nurse stands behind me.

'I think I've got the wrong place.'

'Who are you looking for?' She goes back to the desk, and opens her register.

'No one.' And then I realise how foolish that sounds. 'I mean – he's not here anyway.' And that sounds worse. I feel myself blushing.

I glance again into the room. There is the painting of Sydney.

The nurse smiles. 'If you wait, he'll be along soon.'

'No. I was looking for someone else. I know where I am now. Thank you.' I rush quickly back down the corridor, towards the lifts.

I wait for the lift. Tears fill my eyes. I hear sounds behind me and I turn around.

A gaunt young man with purple sores on his face is shuffling along, leaning on his friend who looks at me mournfully. The young man looks at me too. He has large eyes and a gentle smile. They move on down the corridor.

The lift opens. I rest my forehead against its cold wall. Outside, the afternoon sun is beating down. I step out through the gates and look back once. It's all right.

Three o'clock on the Sunday morning. Matteo and I lie awake talking, our feet sore from dancing. In the darkness, we can just make out the safe sex poster hanging on his door.

'I went to the hospice today.'

A pause. 'I've missed him so much at times, Maria. I owe him a great deal.'

We lie silently for a little longer, listening to each other's breathing. Matteo speaks. 'I hope we live to compare each other's dentures. And have sword-fights with our walking-sticks.'

It was difficult to grasp that, as we sat at Kevin's place, Jon's body was wrapped in plastic in the hospice morgue.

With a bottle of red wine and fresh buttered bread, we sat and toasted him. We sprawled on the carpet, on the sofas, eating and drinking while the mid-morning urban sounds started up.

'I'm going to say something at the funeral,' Robbo said. 'I'm going to speak about him the way I knew him.' The strength in his voice stunned us.

'I'm not staying for the funeral,' I said. 'I've said goodbye to Jon. But I'll write something if you'll read it out.' Robbo nodded.

We decided to sleep away the exhaustion in the afternoon, to let our minds switch off.

Before lying down, I wrote something for the funeral. 'Jon is someone I was proud to call my friend. He brought out the best in people, gave so much support and laughter. I only have one regret. I would've loved my baby daughter to have grown up loving and learning from her Uncle Jon. But I taught him something too. There is no such thing as a typical Italian woman, just as there is no typical gay man or lesbian. I was there holding his hand when he found out about his illness. I was there holding his hand when he died. I'll hold his hand again when God reunites us.'

I read over my words. Were they insensitively proclaiming what Jon's parents and many of the congregation might not want to hear? 'I don't know why I was born this way. I just am this way,' Jon would often say. 'So only my Creator knows what all this is about.' The people at the funeral would be praying to that Creator. Jon's parents seemed to have accepted that his sexuality was certainly out of their parental hands, not for them to condemn even if they couldn't condone it. I thought about Christ's teachings, and the way humanity is selective in its interpretations. I decided to leave my funeral note as it was.

In early March, I received a card from Jon's parents. 'Thank you so very much for being such a good and true friend to our son. May God richly bless you. We shall always remember with gratitude your love and most especially your support on that last night. We can never thank you enough.'

I wished them well.

Kevin and I go walking on Monday. I am to leave that afternoon. We go to a coffee shop, sit near a window. The sun streams in, lighting Kevin's face. Yesterday, Robbo graduated from his nursing studies, and we discuss the ceremony.

Kevin tells me how well things are working out with Terry. We talk about his work nursing AIDS patients and counselling their families and friends. We talk about my teaching and studies, swap anecdotes about family-members and friends. We reflect on the day in August when I had driven to school with the strange sensation I would see Kevin. And there he stood in the main office.

'Your working year soon came to an end, and in a couple of weeks, another will begin,' he muses. 'Does anyone ever mention Jon?'

'Now and again. When we reminisce. When we dare to admit that it hasn't been the same.'

'It was quite a drama that you confronted them with at the beginning of last year, wasn't it?'

I nod and stir my chocolate with my straw.

Monday morning routines perched uncomfortably on my shoulders, but I had a job to do.

I drove to work calmly, until, as I neared the school, I glanced to the right to where the balcony of Jon's first house hovered over tree-tops. The principal beckoned me to his office, and he and Peter sat silently, waiting for me to speak.

They understood and would explain to the School Board if necessary. Peter called the staff together and told them the truth firmly and compassionately. I stood near the back wall where I could see everyone. Afterwards I was hugged and comforted, but I couldn't help wishing the hugs and comfort could've been for Jon when he needed them.

Kevin sent a letter for the staff, and thanked them for the support and friendship shown to Jon. 'He wanted to be closer to many of you but unfortunately a gay way of life is not often accepted within a school and he feared discrimination. I ask you to remember him for who he was.' I walked past that letter everyday for two weeks and smiled.

Graduation weekend Kevin, Robbo and I reflect, as they drive me to the bus-station. The three of us together again, huddled in the front seat. The parting is difficult, as it was when I left after Jon's death.

The bus-station is cheerful. People smile. That suits me. I feel very much alive. The airport had been grim. Nobody had smiled. That had suited me.

As the bus begins its long road back to Adelaide, I feel a sense of exhilaration and release, just as I had felt as the plane lifted into the blue sky.

What thoughts filled me then, fill me again now, as if the tapestry is becoming more intricate, but more definite. This is the turning-point, the one Jon said was etched in my palm. There is a task ahead.

The bus rolls into the Adelaide bus-station. I want to hurry out. For there, waiting for me, is my life, and there is another smile of love, and in his arms is the smile of innocence and immortality.

I never did like Sydney. Now I know why.

AUTHOR'S NOTE

The publishing of this book has also been an incredible journey. From my secret scribblings soon after Jon's death, seeking release by putting on paper what raced in my mind, to family and friends refusing to let it lie silently on my shelf, to people I'd never known taking it upon themselves to work on my self-doubts and push for its publication, it's been an inspirational journey of networking and faith. It is also a celebration of how unity in diversity is possible in this world of ours that insists on separating us under sexual, social, racial, political, religious labels.

How do I begin to thank everyone and run the risk of forgetting someone?

To Kevin and Robbo, with gratitude and respect, and to Jon's old friends, Gary and Linda, Jenny and others who have their own stories to tell. Thank you for allowing our subjective interpretations to be told.

To Rob, my best friend and partner. If only all heterosexual men were like you.

To Stephanie, for patience shown when her Mammà was glued to the computer for days, and for the refreshing intervals of play and laughter.

To my family, for encouragement and support. In particular, my parents, Dora and Stefano, who taught me the basics in life rather than confuse me with unnecessary complexities.

To friends, old and new, gay, lesbian and straight, of diverse cultural, social and political backgrounds, who stood by me, shared their own stories, and never cease to overwhelm me with their strength in the face of many obstacles. In particular, Maria and Mike, Matteo, Maurice and Elena,

Maria A., Chris Rillo, Patricia and Gianni, Connie, Lucy and Mario, Silvana, Lina, Soulla, Malloy, Jyanni, Andrew, John, John, Alan, Tim, Kenton and Michael, Roberto, Andrew, Maria, S, L and D, G and S, Tony, C., Wayne.

To my three guardian angels: Elizabeth Mansutti, Malcolm Cowan and Ian Purcell. Three dynamic people who work for social justice, who found time to listen to my ramblings and whom I could always turn to for advice. I admire your insights, energy, and strength of conviction.

To the eighty members of the Uranian Society for gay men present at my reading and discussion on 30 September, 1990. You'll never know how important was your willingness to listen to this nervous woman trying to tell you about things you live with every day. That evening gave me the final sense of conviction and purpose to commit myself to this project.

To the members of the Catholic church group 'Acceptance' for gay men and lesbians and their allies, and to their chaplain, Fr Maurice Shinnick, for his affirmation of my project.

To leaders within the Catholic Education Office in Adelaide who have supported me.

To colleagues at work who were Jon's friends, and who have stood by me. In particular, Jim and Katrina, Michael and Simone, Mary, Peter, Bill, Neta and Fr Bernie Crawford.

To Jane Arms, the editor, and to Michael Bollen the publisher.

And to many others: friends, colleagues and 'experts' of one kind or another, such as Dr Kay Schaffer, Mick Bocchino; Fathers Lawrie MacNamara, Michael Trainer, and Kevin Penry; Geraldine Rice, Sr Meg, Lina Ferraro, Myra Betschild, who took the time to encourage me, read my manuscript, or talk to me about so many of the issues in this book.

Wakefield Press thanks David Hay and Michael Speers for their gift.